Eat.
Nourish.
Glow.

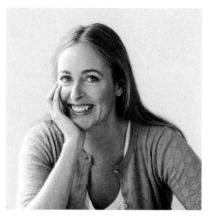

Amelia Freer qualified from The Institute of Optimum Nutrition (ION) in 2007 after a period of 4 years training. She is a member of the British Association for Applied Nutrition and Nutritional Therapy (BANT) and is registered with the Complementary and Natural Healthcare Council (CNHC).

Amelia runs her own thriving London-based clinic, has a home-cooked Freer Food meal delivery service, and a successful track record yielding tangible and dramatic results for her clients. Her clients come to her primarily seeking help with improving energy levels, weight management, cardiovascular health, mental health, digestive wellness and fending off the aging process—or some combination of these. She is vehemently against diets and calorie counting. This is her first book.

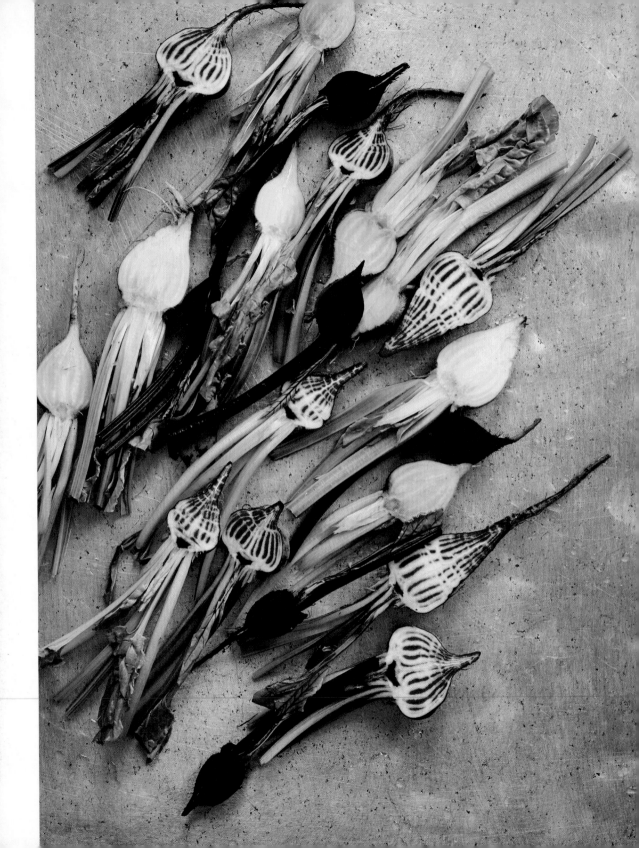

Eat.
Nourish.
Glow.

10 easy steps
for losing weight,
looking younger
and feeling healthier

Amelia Freer

Nutritional therapist and healthy eating expert

HARPER WAVE

An Imprint of HarperCollinsPublishers

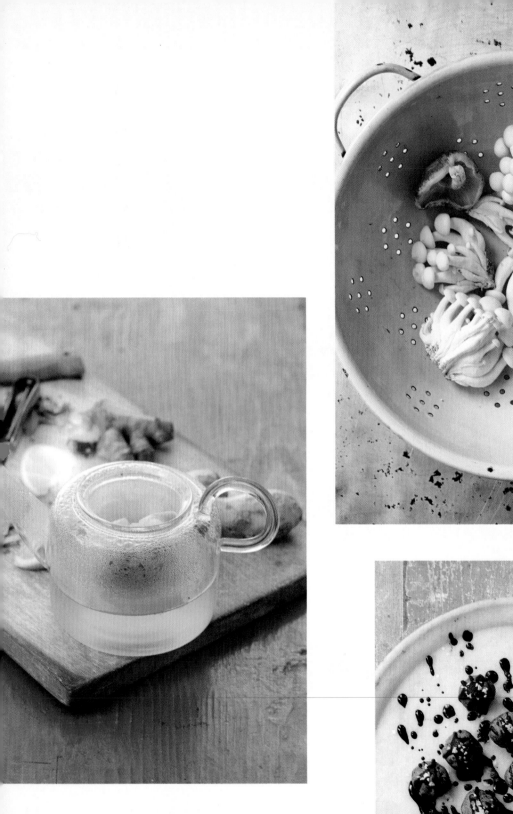
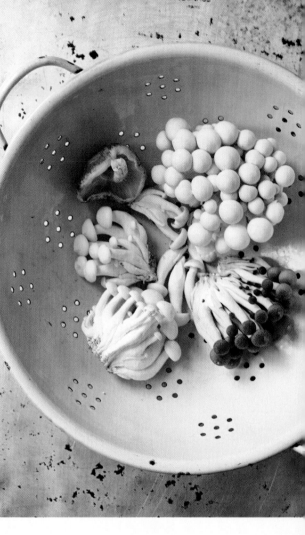
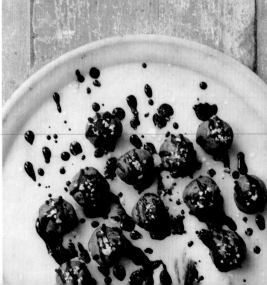

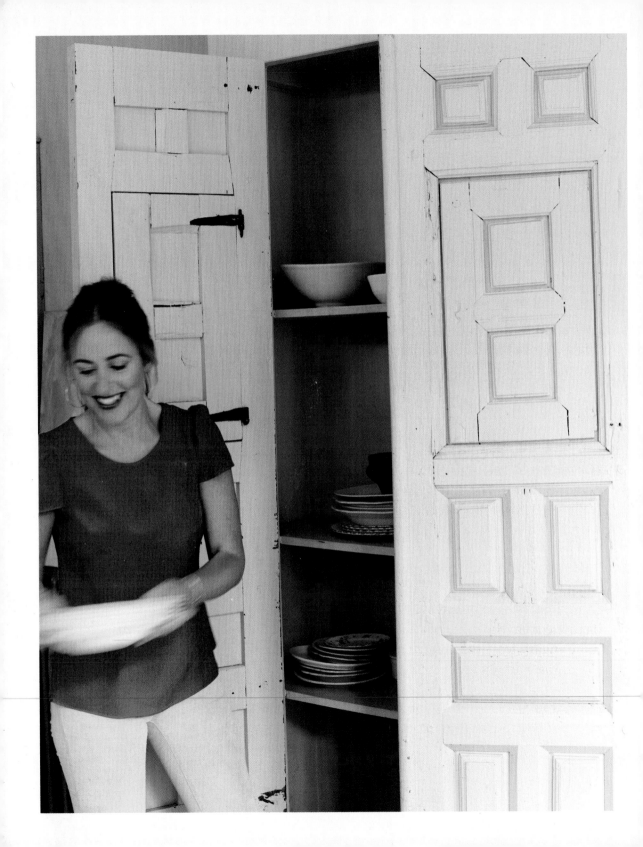

Introduction

Like a lot of people my age I was brought up in a household where my mum cooked our evening meals from scratch. But like all households, we resorted to the standard breakfasts of cereal or toast, and lunch was at school. I was slim and healthy as a child, but as a teenager I developed terrible acne and things started to get worse in my early twenties when I moved to London after university.

Back then I just ate for convenience. I didn't think about my food choices, nor link them to how I felt each day. To me, fast food always meant junk food like burgers or takeout, but I was eating just another type of fast food without realizing it in the form of pasta, ready-made meals, croissants and sandwiches. Everything was quick, factory-made, processed and full of wheat, sugar and little else.

I remember waking up feeling tired and groggy, so I drank lots of sugary tea to perk myself up and grabbed a croissant, some toast or a wrap from a local or chain café on my way to work. Lunch was a sandwich or baguette from the same place and I had chocolate in the afternoons—with more sugary tea—to energize me.

I was working as a PA to The Prince of Wales and I loved my job, but it was busy and demanding. I used to arrive home, exhausted (not because of the job it turns out but because of my terrible diet) and couldn't be bothered to cook so I would have cheese on toast or a plate of pasta with a glass of wine while slumped in front of the TV, or I would be out socially, which often involved eating pasta, bread, desserts and drinking wine. I felt rubbish, but day in day out, I made exactly the same food choices without any further thought.

How were my food choices affecting me? Well, I wasn't overweight, but I wasn't healthy either. I felt exhausted all the time. Literally, all the time. I woke up tired, I felt tired all day, especially in the afternoons, and I fell onto my sofa every night feeling tired. I also suffered from terrible irritable bowel syndrome (IBS). My tummy looked and felt like it had a football stuffed inside it most days, and my skin would still break out into what looked like teenage acne. I took quite a few courses of the drug Roaccutane and that's when my body just said enough. Recurrent colds and infections, shingles and low mood took hold. I was a mess!

I bounced from doctor to doctor and tried massage, acupuncture and hypnosis to make myself feel better but nothing helped. Sharing my frustrations with my roommate one evening, who knew a lot about nutrition, she suggested I try cutting down on my wheat, caffeine and sugar habits and encouraged me to see a nutritionist. It felt alien and impossible to me but that first insight from my roommate and the nutritionist I subsequently saw was the start of this incredible journey I have been on ever since.

As the nutritionist explained the effects food can have on how our body functions, a flame lit inside me and I knew I needed to learn about this for myself. At 28 I went back to college, earning a diploma in Nutritional Therapy at The Institute for Optimum Nutrition (ION) for four years. I was nervous being the age I was and starting again, but on the first day I came alive and knew I was in exactly the right place.

It was there that I started to look at food as medicine. Not as something to just quickly eat to keep hunger at bay, but as something that can nourish and protect us, and also help us to get the best out of every day instead of enduring every day as I had been. During the course I made many changes to my diet and began a mission to create meals that matched my new food knowledge and my health needs, but which also tasted great and comforted me in the way my old food habits used to. I hadn't had any fancy training as a chef; I just called it food assembly. I chose the ingredients I knew my body needed and then I chose the flavors. It didn't need to be complicated (see the Toolkits on page 216). For me it was about simplicity, enjoyment, taste and nourishment. I can never force myself to

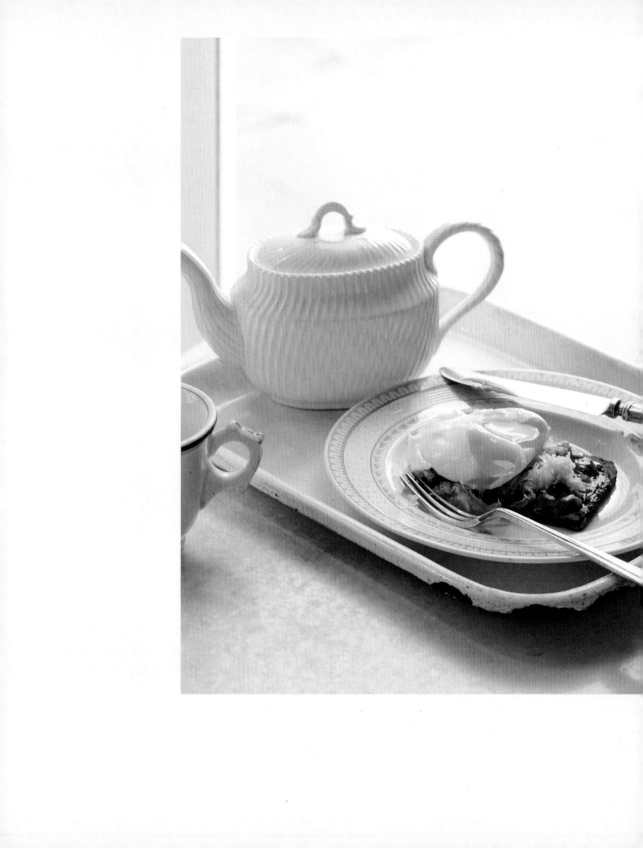

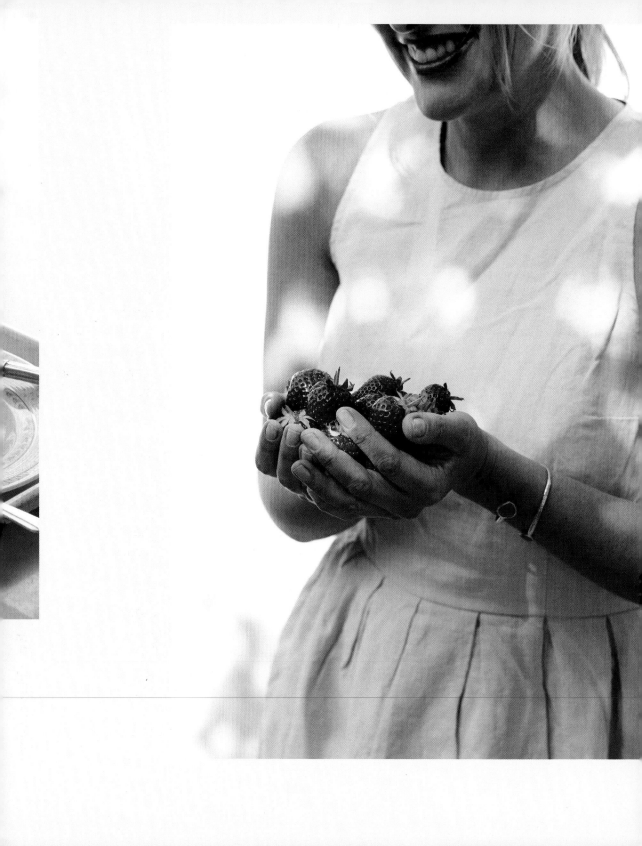

eat anything just because it's healthy. It has to taste great—as the saying goes, "you can lead a horse to water . . ." Once I graduated as a nutritional therapist, I used all my old experiences and new knowledge to help my clients. I know how many of you will be feeling as you read this book and attempt to make changes to your own diet, as I have been there myself. I know how hard it can be to break food habits and get out of your comfort zone at home and socially, but it is possible. As you start to feel the benefits you will want to make more changes to your diet and lifestyle.

That was over 10 years ago and over that time my health has improved dramatically. My original practice in the North of England and my current practice in London have grown and thrived. I continue to study and learn as scientific research constantly evolves in nutrition and health, so I keep abreast of the information and trends and then adapt my knowledge to meet my clients' needs. Oh boy, has my knowledge changed, and I know about the confusion and frustration that many people can feel about the constant fads and changing messages coming from the diet and nutrition industries. Sometimes I go to lectures and learn something new that makes my tummy turn as I realize it conflicts with what I was originally taught and what I have told clients in the past, but I love how rapidly and dramatically this area is growing and how more than ever before, nutrition and nutritional therapy are getting the much-deserved attention they deserve. No longer are we focusing only on cures but now we want to know how to prevent the major illnesses of today. Instead of waiting to be fixed, we want to know how not to get "broken" in the first place. There is still a long way to go but I want to share some of the information and practices I have gathered over my journey to better health with you in this book.

I continue to advance my studies and I'm fortunate enough to be currently studying at the Institute for Functional Medicine (IFM) in the United States. I completed my initial five days of training with them in 2011 on how to apply the principles of functional medicine in clinical practice and I now work with all my clients through this practice, which is a patient-centered and holistic approach to healthcare. No two people are the same and no two treatments or optimum diets are alike. However, there are guidelines that can apply to anyone and I use these to inform the 10 Principles outlined in the book.

Most notably, through my own experience of working with clients, I have learned that knowing the science is not enough. I have learned that each person that sits in front of me has their own unique health and life story. In order to accurately advise them, I must understand them and their journey, understand all the factors that influence their ability to make better choices when selecting their food and understand their emotional relationship with food as well as working hard to identify the underlying causes of their symptoms. Many want a quick fix and think it's so easy for me to tell everyone what "the perfect diet" is or what the "best" supplements are to take. We are all individual and there is not one right diet for everyone. It took me quite a long time of experimenting and improving my diet over the years to get it right for me, so that I can be symptom free and feel my best. What I can say for sure is that eating food in its most natural form is the very best place to start. I have written this book with the hope that it helps you to become more conscious about the food choices you make and connect them to your health, and learn how to make changes to your diet for the long term. This book isn't a personal approach to your health, but I hope that it gives you the experience of working with a nutritional therapist such as myself, covering the most important areas that I have found essential to address with each of my clients.

Every time you think, "I can't do that" or "I don't have time to eat like that," just think that I thought that as well at one stage, but I did make the changes and you know what? They were actually much easier than I thought, and the results were amazing. I can't imagine going back to my old eating habits. I don't miss them or feel like I'm missing out. If anything I was missing out back then because I was living a half-life of feeling tired and sluggish. So read this book, know you can make the changes and believe in yourself because if I can do it, so can you.

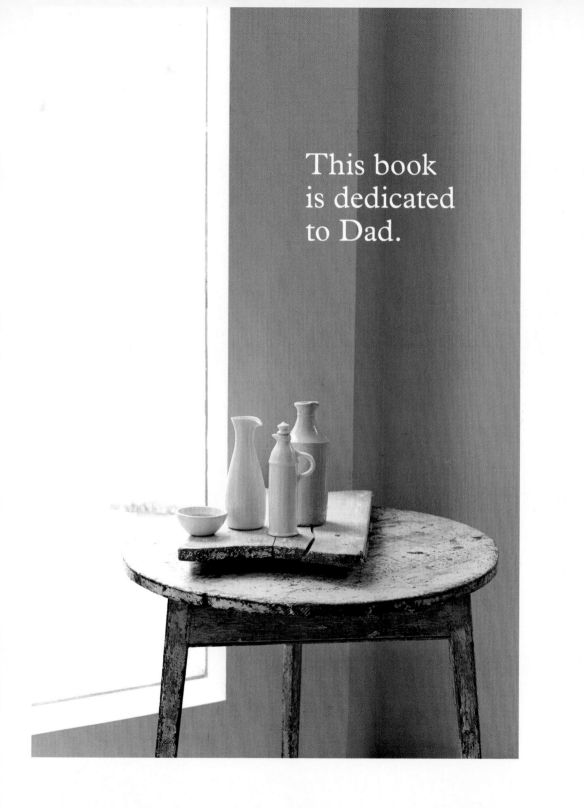

This book
is dedicated
to Dad.

Eat. Nourish. Glow.

So what should you start with? / Still confused? Keep a two-week food diary / Sugar / Gluten / Alcohol / Dairy / Caffeine / Listen to your gut

Just one thing.

—No. 1

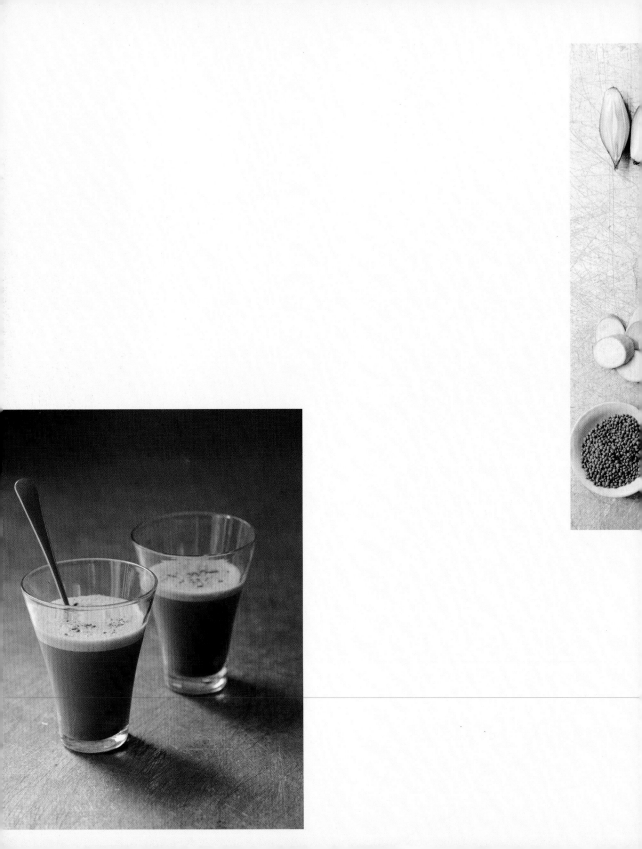

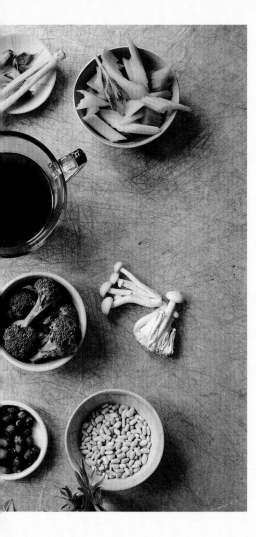
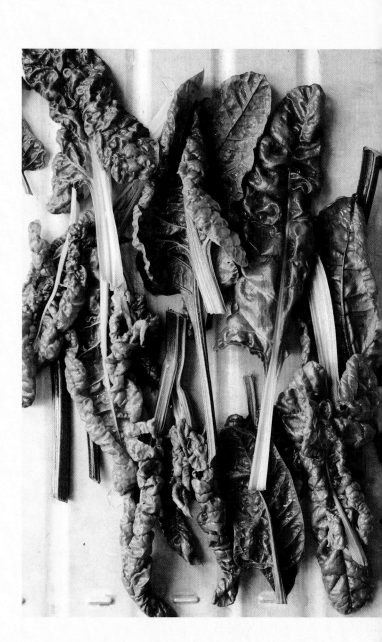

"Listen to your body. It's smarter than you."

Let's start at the beginning. As an eager and newly graduated nutritional therapist, I ventured out into the clinical world bursting with knowledge and passion. Having committed my head and heart to four years learning the exact, precise and *perfect* way to eat to be healthy, I assumed that everyone wanted to know what I knew. What a fright I got! They didn't. Most wanted quick fixes with life-changing results. As a student I was highly trained in how to work with clients, helping them to change their diets, but still, my passion took over and in the early days my poor clients would leave feeling overwhelmed and frightened, with lists and pages of handouts and I would be buzzing having imparted all I knew. Not quite as inspiring as I had hoped it turned out—all I had actually done was set them up for failure by setting the bar way too high. My thinking came from a good place. I had managed to transform my own health through making changes to my diet with amazing results and so I wanted everyone to have the same experience as me.

I learned quickly that there was a far bigger picture that I needed to observe. It wasn't about me or my journey, I needed to really understand the person sitting in front of me—their lifestyle, their relationship with food, their confidence and their diet weaknesses or preferences.

Everybody has their own story with food and getting it right is far more complex than being given the information. I find that some clients just need an update about food and want facts and knowledge so they can make smart choices; others need a nudge in the right direction; some need me to carefully hold their hand as I teach them how to introduce new foods and habits while weaning themselves off addictive foods, while there are others who fear food and have yoyo dieted for years and need help in slowly unpicking the web of nutritional confusion that has robbed them of their enjoyment of food. Some of my clients simply have bad food habits and don't know it, or they do know it but don't know how to change. There are a million different stories and complexities that can factor in how we choose to eat that go way beyond calories!

And people don't like to fail—they will often give up before they fully start. If you are fairly unfit and decide to run a marathon, it might not happen, but if you sign up for a mile, you will be more likely to give it a go, and the 5k, 10k and half marathons might follow. It's the same with eating well—you are far more likely to succeed if you make changes slowly and steadily. Naturally the best kind of healthy eating is the kind that we do long term, not once or twice a year. Being healthy can sometimes feel complicated to begin with, so changing one thing at a time keeps things simple.

This is exactly how I did it. Though I was so hard on myself, I felt totally ashamed and frustrated that I couldn't do it all at once despite knowing it was what I needed to do for my health. I assumed that others could do it and that it was only me who needed to do it bit by bit. If you told me ten years ago I would be eating as healthily as I am now I wouldn't have believed you. Or to be more precise, I wouldn't have believed in myself. When I first explored nutrition I was drinking ten cups of sugary tea a day, eating sandwiches for lunch, cheese, pasta, chocolate, chips, bread and more bread. There's no way I could have given up all those things within a week, so I did it my way; frustratingly slowly for my impatient and perfectionist self, but enough to notice a difference and hence begin a deep and very new connection with food and my health. By changing my eating habits little by little, by creating one healthy habit at a time and learning what works for me, I now have a great diet. It certainly didn't happen overnight and this is why I feel so strongly that crash or faddy diets are so damaging. I see this damage with my clients who are trapped in a negative cycle of wanting to eat better, feel slim and vibrant but not being able to cope with the restrictions while living busy lives. So just as with me, I came to realize that slow and steady really does win the health race after all.

I stopped asking my clients to give up everything they loved (or *thought* they loved—more on this later!) and instead asked them to let go of just one thing and focus on all of the things to *include* in their diets—a far more positive approach and it worked. Nearly all of them found they could do this fairly easily and once they started to see and feel the positivity, they were keen to keep going. And so it went on. By giving them small goals, instead of a huge mountain to climb, they found it easy and felt proud of their achievements, which spurred them on. The results were and still are astounding—from improved energy, better sleep, clearer skin, losing weight, better bowels, focused thinking, less pain, brighter moods AND their taste buds started to change, the sugar cravings diminished and suddenly it wasn't such a battle to make healthier choices, and keep them.

Now, I really love food and I feel that everyone should be able to love food. However, the foods that I used to think I loved are no longer what I would have at the top of my list. In fact, I would feel pretty annoyed if I was forced to eat those things now. My love of food is still present but my tastes and choices have drastically changed along the way. I don't feel hungry or deprived and I never stress or feel guilty about food. I'm never on a diet. I just learned how to eat in a way that makes me feel and look better, which I then passed on to my clients, and now I'm going to share this with you too . . .

> ## "Your life does not get better by chance, it gets better by change."

Jim Rohn

So what should you start with?

This is for you to decide, but it might help if you recognize yourself in some of the clients I have met over the years.

The working mum A working mum of two young children came to see me feeling overweight, sluggish and numb with tiredness. It was affecting how she parented, how she worked, her confidence and how she interacted with her friends and family. She knew she was tired from working four days a week and looking after two young children but she was sure she shouldn't be feeling *this* tired. Sound familiar? She had had a checkup with her GP and there was nothing medically wrong to cause these symptoms. She said a sentence that I hear a lot! "I know what I should eat and my diet is pretty healthy." Her diet consisted of store-bought meals and although expensive and "good quality," the reality was that they were high in sugar, carbs and not at all fresh, so lacking in essential nutrients. From looking at her food diary, I could understand why she wasn't feeling her best. Her breakfast was usually granola, yogurt and fruit compote from a chain coffee shop near where she worked. Lunch was a sandwich from the same place. Dinner was a ready-made meal from a good supermarket picked up on the way home—usually something like a fish pie or lasagne with salad. All her meals contained vegetables or fruits and came from good places, so she figured she was eating healthily. She also relied on several coffees and the "occasional" cookie or cake to get her through the day. Once I highlighted with a pen, just how much of her diet each day was one form of sugar or another, she started to see just how lacking her diet actually was.

Trust me, when you get into this habit the mental fog and tiredness will lift, the flab around your waist will fall off and you will wonder why on earth you didn't do this sooner.

So I suggested that her "one" thing to give up was ready-made meals and instead to focus on preparing her own food. After all, she didn't feed ready-made meals to her kids, so we worked out meals that she could make for everyone and cut out the store-bought stuff. Her biggest resistance to my suggestion was lack of time. My goodness is that a common line? It's one of the biggest excuses for not eating properly. And I get it—but only to a point. When I dug a little deeper I realized she did have time, she wasn't using it properly and she wasn't prepared. Many of you reading this are probably nodding along because you don't have enough time either, right? But ask yourself this—how much time do you spend on the sofa every evening browsing on your phone or laptop? How much time do you spend watching TV when the kids are in bed or when you get home from work? I have clients who say they are too busy to cook and they rely on ready-made meals, but they eat those ready-made meals in front of an hour-long cooking show.

If you have time to watch those shows you have time to cook—cook more, watch TV less. Trust me, when you get into this habit the mental fog and tiredness will lift, the flab around your waist will fall off and you will wonder why on earth you didn't do this sooner. I'm not talking about gourmet feasts but more about food assembly. It just doesn't need to be complex or fancy, just real. At the back of this book I have included a few quick and easy recipes that I regularly throw together in minutes, so don't assume that good food involves a lot of time and effort and that ready-made meals or shortcut staples like pasta with sauce from a jar are the only way. I'm going to show you how to make very easy healthy meals in minutes. I'm not a chef and I often don't get my cooking right, but I can throw a few simple meals together that taste great and are fantastically healthy. I have spent years giving clients alternatives to all their favorite meals and I'm going to do the same for you.

Back to my client. To ease her in, I suggested she make just one of her meals from scratch. I also gave her lots of ideas for breakfasts, lunches and dinners that took minutes to prepare and also suggestions of the healthiest fast food options. She started making dinner every night, which took the same amount of time to put on the plate as the microwave meals she had been relying on. She made large batches and took the leftovers in to work for lunch the next day. Last, she started making her own breakfasts to take to work that were simple and quick and took less time to prepare than standing in the line for her overpriced, sugary granola. The changes were rapid. Her energy started to improve and she started to feel less bloated and stressed. She really enjoyed her new routine and reconnecting with cooking. Within two months she had lost 14 pounds and the mental fog and tiredness lifted. She gave up just one thing—ready-made meals—yet the change was huge.

"The 80s Dieter" Then there is "The 80s Dieter." This way of eating was huge in the Eighties and Nineties and many of these dieters picked up their habits from their mothers who ate this way throughout their childhoods in a bid to stay slim. The "80s Dieter" knows everything about calories but nothing about nutrition. They avoid fat but their diets are soaked in sugar, which causes them to gain weight and feel awful (I will explain more about this in Chapter Six). They buy diet foods and soft drinks, count calories and watch the scales. Sometimes they are thin but not at all healthy and suffer a wide range of symptoms. A good diet to them is one that has very little fat and calories in it and results in quick weight loss. They may feel exhausted and hungry a lot of the time, but at least the scales are going down. A typical daily diet consists of fruit and low-fat yogurt for breakfast or a "diet" shake, a baked potato or pasta for lunch, a "diet" microwave meal or fat-free salad for dinner followed by a "diet" mousse or yogurt. Throughout the day they drink diet cola or fruit juice, they take sweeteners in their tea and they treat themselves to a skinny muffin from a coffee shop because the word "skinny" in the name makes them think it's healthy. Let's just get this straight—it's not! Without

them understanding it, their whole diet is sugar-soaked, which can be potentially detrimental to their health. They either have willpower of steel or they fail and give in to the constant cravings and forever yoyo with their weight, feeling hungry and deprived. In their case, I suggest they give up sugar.

The beige "food rut" dieter This is another common client I see. They rely on toast for breakfast, pasta or a sandwich for lunch and more pasta or risotto for dinner. Their whole diet is only one color and a meal without grains or potatoes just doesn't seem right to them. If they have a salad or some soup they need a chunk of bread with it. Many carb addicts assume their diet is OK. After all, they reason that pasta and bread are low in fat and healthy for us, right? But sugars are made from the carbohydrates we eat especially the white processed ones like white bread, white rice and white pasta. Even the brown varieties that look healthy are still processed and still convert to sugar in the body. Our bodies aren't designed to have excess levels of sugar in the bloodstream, which is what happens when we eat these kinds of carbs. The effect on our mood, energy, hunger and weight is plain to see. What is key to understand if this way of eating is resonating with you then I would encourage that the "beige" foods (ie, toast for breakfast, a sandwich for lunch) go and are replaced with colorful vegetables.

Still confused? Keep a two-week food diary

A way to help you decide what you should give up first is to keep a detailed two-week food diary. It helps me to see where my clients are going wrong and it helps them too! For example:

Does your sugary (granola), fat-free (fruit) or carb-only (toast) breakfast cause you to snack constantly before lunch?

Do you rely too much on convenience or packaged food?

Are you falling into the low-fat/high-sugar trap like the "80s Dieter"?

Do you drink wine every night which, as well as being full of sugar, increases your appetite the next day?

Do you severely restrict your calories all day or all week, only to have a blow out in the evening or at the weekend because you are so hungry and fed up with being "good"?

Do you rely on carbs because you think they are easy and quick?

Are you an evening snacker who binges on chocolate and sweets in the hours between finishing dinner and going to bed?

In fact, do your snacks in general let you down?

Take a good look at your food diary, use colored pens to circle different food groups or colors and write down how you feel before and after the foods that feature highly in your diet. You will quickly be able to get to know your relationship with food better and work out your dietary weak spot and the thing you need to give up first.

	Day 1	Day 2	Day 3	Day 4	Day 5	Day 6	Day 7
Breakfast							
Lunch							
Evening meal							
Snacks/ Drinks							
Symptoms/ Feelings							

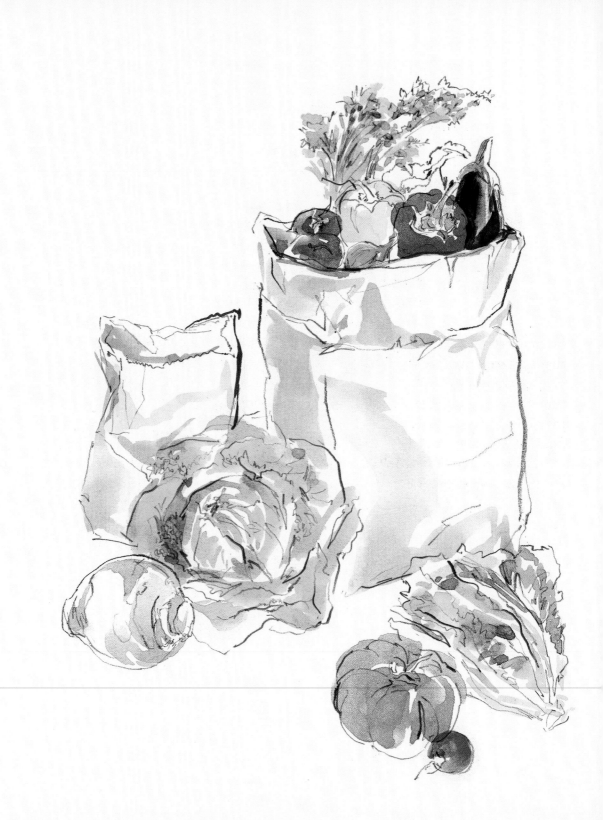

Eat. Nourish. Glow.

> "Food has the power to make or break you. Choose your own destiny."

So my first "one" thing was dairy. I needed to give up so much more but that's where I managed to start. I'm not saying that everyone needs to give up dairy, but I certainly did. And it was hard. Mainly because at that time there were limited alternatives and it was everywhere. But I slowly managed to remove it from my kitchen and my life and it was the starting point of my journey back toward good health.

With clients these days, however, I see a very common triangle of foods that have a boomerang effect, each creating a need for the other—that's Caffeine, Sugar and Alcohol. You will know if this is you. Perhaps one of these foods has a stronger influence in this triangle than the other for you, so that food may be your one thing to give up and get started on the road to better health.

Here are the main foods that ultimately over time are key to address and reduce or remove from your diet, one by one:

Sugar

Why you might give it up I'm a fierce critic of sugar. It's right up there with smoking and drugs and will probably be viewed in a similar way by many in ten years time—I certainly hope so. People used to smoke without any knowledge of the health implications and in a similar way, we have been eating vast amounts of sugar rather blindly, without really knowing if it's OK. And the answer is no it's not.

As a main component of food processing methods, sugar has been corroding our diets and health now for years, despite numerous studies showing how it simply is not compliant with good health. I was in the sugar trap years ago and I see so many clients who are locked into it today. Its impact is detrimental. That's quite a bold statement, but one I stand by.

So, what's wrong with sugar? It's a drug that makes us fat (yes, all those low-fat products are riddled with sugar!) especially around the middle; it creates fat around our organs; it increases our risk of heart disease, cancer and diabetes, and it is now known to contribute to premature aging, and by that I mean anything from wrinkles to Alzheimer's. It's also addictive, both physically and emotionally—studies have shown sugar's effect on the human brain and it has been proven that it is eight times more addictive than cocaine! So don't beat yourself up if you have tried to give it up and failed. For drug addiction, people need to go into rehab and be helped step by step on so many levels. Yet many of us are living with this sugar addiction on a daily basis without the knowledge or support on how to crack it. It's being drip-fed into us, often unknowingly, in so many different forms, but it is possible to break this addiction once you know what and how to eat. I will show you how later on in this book but for now, it's important to be familiar with sugar's role in our health and its many different forms.

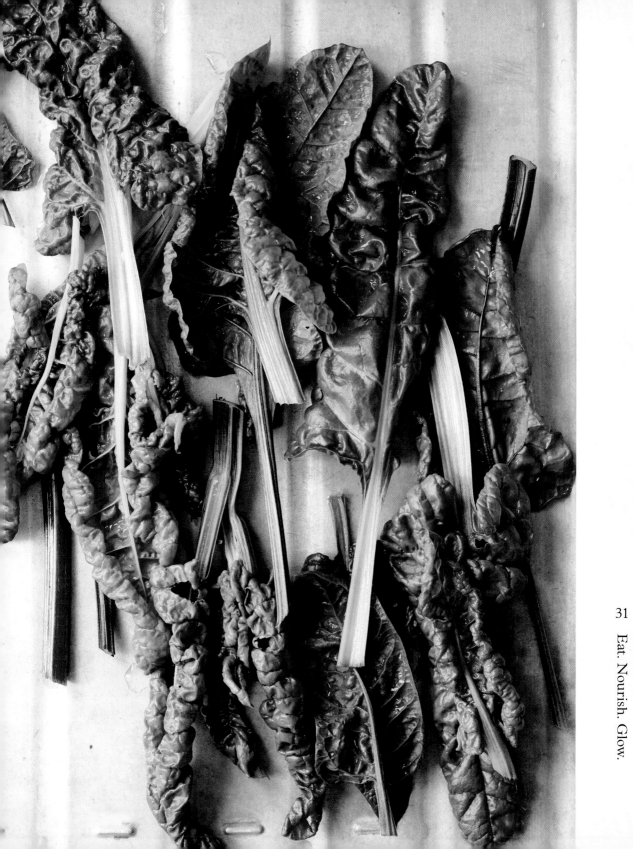

Eat. Nourish. Glow.

I want to keep the science simple but it's important to understand what happens when we eat sugar. Our body is designed to only allow a very small amount of sugar in the bloodstream at any one time—about 1–2 teaspoonfuls. If we eat more than this, the hormone insulin is produced to transport this sugar out of the bloodstream. This sugar, through several mechanisms, gets converted into fat, mainly the kind of fat that gets stored around the waist, but sometimes this can also be "invisible" fat that gets stored around the organs—both are detrimental to our health. If large quantities of sugar are consumed on a regular basis, our cells can become lazy and resistant to the presence of insulin, which increases our risk of some pretty serious diseases like Type 2 diabetes. Increasingly, studies are showing that too much sugar can increase our risk of heart disease, even if we aren't overweight. Excess dietary sugar can also attach itself to our cells and form a hard, sticky crust, a process called glycation. This crust is detrimental to the aging process. When I first start working with clients, I run blood tests to check the levels of sugar and insulin in the blood and look for a specific marker called glycosolated hemaglobin which helps me to identify the client's exposure and management of sugar over the previous three months. These tests are very useful as they help me show clients the damage that sugar could be doing and help motivate them to reduce it.

No matter how much money you spend on amazing skin creams, you simply can't undo the cellular damage that sugar causes from the inside.

To continue with aging. Wrinkles are also the result of glycation—picture a toffee apple or a crème brûlée. Our cells are meant to be soft and plump, like a full water balloon, not hard and caked. No matter how much money you spend on amazing skin creams, you simply can't undo the cellular damage that sugar causes from the inside.

To wrap up my sugar rant, there is an established connection between blood sugar levels and brain health. In August 2013 *The New England Journal of Medicine* reported a study testing the role of this not just for people with diabetes, but with people who consistently have blood sugar elevations.

So are you getting the picture? These are just a few examples of how sugar can negatively impact our health. If you want a trim figure, glowing skin and vibrant energy and not have heart disease, diabetes or a neurological disease, then maybe, you would benefit from addressing how much sugar you are eating.

Sugar in food Cakes, sweets and biscuits are the obvious sources, but it lurks in many other foods, even those that are seemingly healthy—balsamic vinegar, salad dressings, low-fat yogurts, fizzy drinks, fruit juices (even the "healthy" breakfast cartons and the sparkling pastel colored ones that cost a fortune and look so virtuous), breakfast cereals, wine, pasta sauces and ready-made meals. Food manufacturers have been adding it to food for years because it makes food more palatable—and addictive. But that is still only the white powder form. There has been a surge of "sugar-free" treats flooding the market in recent years, but sugar free doesn't always mean sugar free. It means that a sugar substitute has been used—either a chemical version such as aspartame or a natural alternative, such as honey or stevia. Whatever the sweetener, even something as natural as fructose, it still has exactly the same effect on your brain and body. These sweeteners still condition the taste buds to crave sugar, so go easy on them and don't be fooled into thinking that these are better options; even the healthy ones.

I'm still not done . . . ! Whenever we eat a carbohydrate, such as bread, pasta, rice, potatoes, fruit and vegetables, they are all converted into a form of sugar, which enters our bloodstream. Now we make energy from this sugar and we do need some, but we don't need vast quantities and we still want to keep our blood sugar level stable. Vegetables and fruits are the best choices, but even fruit in abundance can be negative if you are also eating lots of the other "sugary" foods. It is so easy to eat too much sugar . . . we are bombarded with it.

How to give it up I'm not going to lie—it's tough! It's a drug. Reducing sugar first starts with understanding it and connecting with how much and what forms you eat it. If you are using sugar, you must be kind but strong with yourself and allow some rehabilitation time. I'm serious. You will never look back. That's not to say you can't ever have a slice of cake or a glass of wine again. I do and of course you will too! I indulge in good red wine with friends and many of my clients have their cake if they want to, but what we are aiming for is to stop the daily drip-feed of sugar in your diet—this simply has to go.

So, how do you give it up? With sugar, total abstinence (to begin with) is the key to breaking the daily addiction that so many of us have. I tell clients to give it up entirely for seven days. And to make the transition easier I suggest some nutritional supplements to help reduce their cravings. Chromium is particularly good for this by helping to keep blood sugar levels stable, which quiets cravings. I also always suggest a source of good-quality protein with every meal, which slows down the release of sugar into the bloodstream and helps to keep us full and hence crave less.

Break sugar associations too. Many of us have grown up seeing sugar as a reward or a comforter. Post-war mums fed their children with jam and honey, which was fairly harmless, because back then children ate home-cooked food like meat and vegetables and sugar was just an occasional treat. There were no processed foods pumped full of additives and sugar; no sugary cereals served up every morning; no plates of pasta or ready-made meals, or unlimited ice creams, chocolate and sweets. The sugar/comfort thing remained and my mother's generation also fed their children cakes as a "treat" or to cheer them up. I was given very sweet tea as a child and as a result, drank endless cups of sugary tea throughout my twenties—especially when I was stressed or tired. If we are weaned on sugar, we tend to turn to these foods as adults when we feel run down, stressed or unhappy. You need to stop seeing sugar as a treat and see it as something that's making you fat, tired and miserable, and if eaten regularly and long term, the cause of serious illness.

Last, be prepared. In the next chapter I talk about how to prepare your house for eating well. We often turn to sugar when we haven't had a proper lunch because there's little food in the fridge, or if we have run out the door and skipped breakfast. It's very important to eat regularly when you are giving up sugar because if you miss a meal and your blood sugar levels drop—or you become hungry—the quick burst of energy and taste that a chocolate bar or biscuit provides proves very tempting.

Gluten

Why you might give it up The term "gluten-free" is suddenly
everywhere. From Hollywood stars to world-class tennis players, and now,
most likely the person sitting next to you at work, everyone is trying it. Many
say it's a fad. But I don't think so; I think gluten-free living is here to stay.

Gluten is a protein present in wheat, rye and barley, so basically it
constitutes a standard breakfast. But its reach is far more than that. It is
present in more than your daily bread—hidden in pre-packaged foods,
sauces, prescription medications, supplements, toothpaste and make-up.
Even foods that are naturally gluten-free or claiming to be gluten-free can
become cross-contaminated in the manufacturing process. Many people
consider that gluten is only a problem for those with celiac disease, but it's
not quite the case.

Celiac disease (CD) is an autoimmune condition that is triggered
by the consumption of gluten and leads to damage and inflammation of
the lining of the digestive tract. People with CD are required to strictly
avoid all sources of gluten. However, it is far more prevalent than was
once thought. Researchers now accept that CD has the capacity to affect
any organ in the body, not just the gut, and it is now believed to be the
most common and neglected life-long genetic disorder in both Europe
and the United States. Originally considered to be exclusively a disease
of the gastrointestinal system, researchers now understand that it's more
common for patients to present without any digestive symptoms, but a
myriad of different health issues including fatigue, infertility, cancer,
rheumatoid arthritis and schizophrenia to name just a few, and it can
present at any age. A list of over 50 diseases that can be caused by eating
gluten was presented in a review paper in *The New England Journal of
Medicine* in 2002. A recent study from Nottingham University found
that almost half a million people in the U.K. have CD without realizing
it—possibly because they aren't presenting classic symptoms or being
accurately tested. Gluten does need to be consumed in order to get an
accurate test for CD.

But CD is just the start . . . Dr. Alessio Fasano, a world-renowned
expert on CD and a professor of pediatrics, medicine and physiology
at the University of Maryland School of Medicine in the U.S. confirms

Dr. Alessio Fasano, a world-renowned expert on CD and a professor of pediatrics, medicine and physiology at the University of Maryland School of Medicine in the U.S. confirms that "the human body cannot digest gluten."

that "the human body cannot digest gluten." That means all of us and this inability to digest it can cause a series of reactions. Our bodies do their best to communicate with us by sending us symptoms and signals, so many people do detect that they may react to gluten because they get bloating, nausea or irritable bowel syndrome (IBS) type symptoms. But gluten is an evasive protein and its effects can be silent.

Giving up wheat isn't such a new trend; many have done it and felt better for it, but being gluten-free is still quite new. This is because a relatively new, but significant term known as non-celiac gluten sensitivity (NCGS) is now causing a rumble. Certainly wheat has been acknowledged as causing issues for many people over the last few years and for some, it can stop at wheat. For others, however, all of the glutinous grains can be problematic, so now researchers have started to delve into this uncharted territory.

Why is there so little awareness of the damaging effects of gluten? I'm told it takes 17 years for scientific knowledge to filter down into mainstream medicine. And certainly in the field of food and science, a lot of the theories are scoffed at, just like sugar, until overwhelming evidence convinces people otherwise.

Unlike sugar—which is increasingly, and quite rightly, being held up as a real health baddie in the national press, there is still little awareness about the potential negative effects of gluten on our health. It was the last thing to go for me. I first cut out wheat years ago, after dairy, but I continued to eat gluten quite unaware it was still contributing to my sluggish and foggy head. I gave it up completely in 2011 and it was one of the best things I have ever done for my health. My real education on the potential risks of eating gluten came from Dr. Tom O'Bryan in 2011. At his first lecture in the U.K., Dr. O'Bryan produced study after study showing the wide-reaching implications of gluten on a vast array of diseases. I left the lecture vowing never to eat gluten again, as his information was so convincing. The transformation to my mind and body after I gave it up was like night and day—it was the final thing that I needed to remove from my diet to really fix my digestive problems and lose that cotton wool feeling in my head. I felt better than I thought I could.

Nutritional experts have been talking about the negative effects of sugar for years, but only very recently has this message been taken seriously and ended up as headlines in the national press. At the beginning of 2014, the World Health Organization drafted guidelines about sugar consumption in the same way it did regarding salt and fat consumption many years previously. It's my view that in a few years time gluten will be held up in the same way. It's not that all gluten is bad for us, but bad gluten is bad for us! Due to manufacturing methods as well as increased availability and consumption, increasing numbers of people are suffering because of the huge amount of gluten in their diet. Awareness is starting to grow, and while going gluten-free has the potential to sound like a fad, there is so much more to it, and it will become mainstream in time.

So as dynamic as it may be in the kitchen, gluten can wreak havoc on our health for some of us, so it might be worth considering if eating gluten is actually a good thing for you or not. Try it and see, but always under the guidance of a qualified nutritional therapist who can help you with the necessary digestive support along the way.

Don't just assume that giving up gluten is only for those with IBS. If you suffer from frequent and unexplained fatigue, head fog, eczema, asthma, joint pain or if you know that you are predisposed to specific autoimmune conditions, then maybe it's worth trying a period without eating gluten and see how you feel.

How to give it up Rather than browsing in the "gluten-free" aisle in the supermarket, opt for foods that are naturally gluten-free. Crunchy salads, poached eggs, nuts, seeds, salmon steak, poultry or succulent prawns for instance. Focus on all the delicious foods that you can eat rather than worrying about what you will be giving up. Gluten-free products can be so misleading—just because they are gluten-free does not mean that they are good for you and usually they are filled with sugar and preservatives, so read the labels and see what they actually contain instead of gluten.

In terms of what to avoid, gluten is found in wheat, barley and rye, which means most breakfast cereals, most breads, pasta, cakes, muffins and beer. Because it's used as a binder, it's also found in soy sauce, dressings and sauces like tomato sauce and salad dressing—read the labels carefully as it's everywhere!

Again, preparation is vital. Don't just have bags of pasta and bread in your house because you will fall back on them when you are hungry. Stock up on lots of naturally gluten-free foods (I'll talk more about which ones to buy in Chapter Two).

Alcohol

Why you might give it up We all know that alcohol derails us physically and emotionally if consumed in excess, and it is another drug for many. If you don't rely on alcohol and drink sensibly, then you don't need to cut it out altogether. But many of my clients seem to have a blind spot when it comes to alcohol. They would never dream of eating a chocolate bar but they will easily drink a whole bottle of wine with a friend after work or have several glasses every evening, which contains more sugar than the chocolate bar. Alcohol is absorbed directly through the stomach lining and stimulates the production of a neurotransmittor called GABA which has a calming effect on us—no wonder we use it to unwind at the end of a busy day. It also leads to huge blood sugar fluctuations which directly impacts our energy levels, our food choices and naturally our waistline due to the sugar content in most alcohols or the mixers we use, and the foods that we eat while drinking and the next day.

Alcohol also needs to be processed by the liver and it is a well known fact that it causes a strain on liver health if consumed in excess. The Government safety standard for alcohol consumption is 14 units per week for women and 21 units for men. One unit is ½ oz. of pure alcohol or the old-fashioned standard wine glass. The large 8-oz. glasses we now tend to drink can be the equivalent of three units so if you have two or three glasses you can see how easy it is to go above the weekly safety limit. For more information visit www.niaaa.nih.gov/alcohol-health/overview-alcohol-consumption/moderate-binge-drinking.

How to give it up If you know that you have a real problem with alcohol I strongly urge you to see your GP to get the appropriate help as it can wreak havoc on your health as well as destroy your relationships and working life. If you think you probably drink a little too much and want to work on improving your health, the best way is abstinence. Choose a period of time and find alternative drinks and activities to fill in the times when you might normally unwind with a glass of wine or beer. When many of my clients first come to see me they drink one or several glasses of wine a night. It often starts as a way to relax then it becomes a habit and something to associate with unwinding for the night. So break that association and find another way to relax. Going forward, you can enjoy wine occasionally but set up a structure to avoid it becoming a nightly habit because it will take a toll on your body, waistline and energy levels. If you lead a busy social life then try alternating the nights you drink or choose two nights per week when you can drink.

Dairy

Why you might give it up We are all individuals, and while cow's milk is supposed to be for baby calves, we humans have been consuming it for thousands of years. But at what cost to our health? Personally when I consume dairy produce, my acne returns, my belly bloats, my menstrual cycle gets confused and I get frequent sinus issues and headaches. Not so nice and while I used to love cheese, I seriously think twice before I eat it if I'm prepared to endure the following two weeks post eating it! But to each his own. Many people say they are fine eating dairy despite being riddled with eczema, rosacea, sinusitis, IBS, joint pain and headaches to name a few. Of course, we have no way to prove that dairy is the cause but hey, it would be nice not to live with those conditions . . . surely? And maybe, cutting out dairy might help? Surely it's worth a try. Yes I know that the calcium question will come up. I have been dairy free for almost 15 years and the last time I had my calcium levels tested they were perfectly normal. Some of us can cope with cow's milk, but for many it can lead to inflammation, which shows itself in conditions like asthma, eczema, acne and hormonal imbalances. It can also make you bloated. In addition, it's now not such a pure product due to mass production, chemicals and hormones. So if you do drink milk or eat cream or cheese, at least buy organic.

How to give it up It's never been easier to give up dairy. When I gave it up 15 years ago there were few options. Soy became a trendy alternative in the Nineties, but it has estrogenic properties and is genetically modified now. In the past it's been cited as being beneficial in some instances for supporting female hormonal health due to its estrogenic properties, but now it seems to cause more food intolerances. I think our diets are so much higher in dairy in the U.K. that we get too much estrogen from dairy and meat as it is. So if you do use soy, buy organic and don't have it in large quantities.

Alternatives to dairy There are now such a wide variety of great healthy alternatives. I suggest my clients try nut milks such as almond or cashew and coconut milk, all of which are now widely available. Butter is a great health product for those that can eat it and ghee is an excellent fat to cook with and usually suitable for sensitive individuals (sadly not me). So if butter isn't OK for you then try using coconut butter instead, but definitely avoid the plastic tub spreads. As for other calcium sources, you can get it from food. We have been led to believe that we can only get calcium from dairy sources, but in fact it is widely available in other foods, especially if we are eating a natural diet and in particular, dark green leafy vegetables, which are a rich source of calcium. So if you juice them, mash them, blend them or steam them, calcium is just one of the many reasons to eat your greens.

Caffeine

Why you should give it up There are many reported health benefits to caffeine and so I am not at all anti it nor tell my clients to give it up, as I think I would be out of work. Personally, I am rather new to drinking coffee but I have enjoyed tea all of my life. What is important to understand about caffeine is that we can use it for its benefits in the right

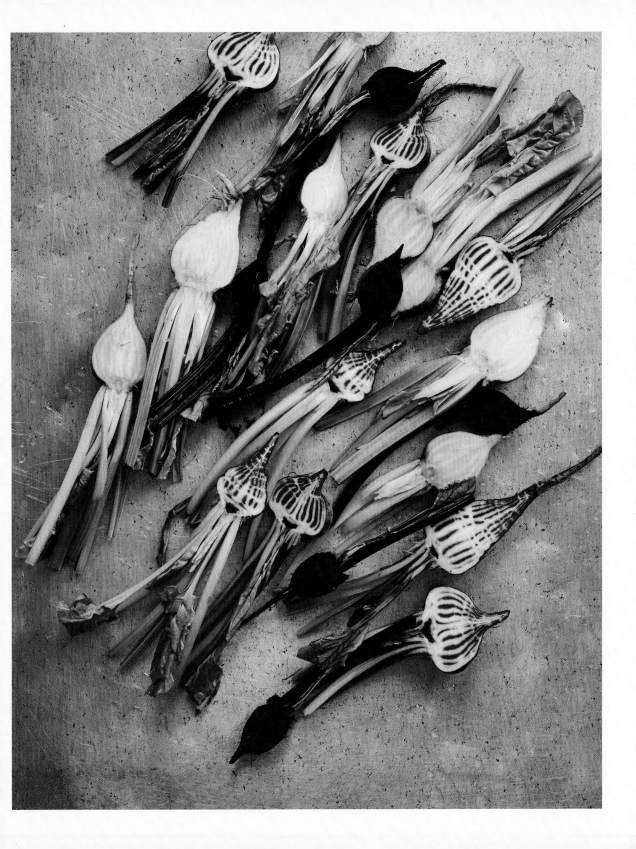

way or we can use it with incredibly negative effects. I drink one or two cups of organic, freshly made black coffee with a spoonful of coconut butter blended in every day. This provides me with the antioxidants and the energy release, but the oil stops me from getting the insulin high that can set us off on that blood sugar rollercoaster all day. I never drink it after lunch as I need to have good-quality sleep each night and caffeine is known for its stimulating effects, which can disrupt sleep in sensitive individuals.

How to give it up I find with my clients that their overuse of coffee is something else that they need to break, like their post-work wine or post-dinner sugar binge. They love the ritual of making coffee when they wake up or buying it on their way to work. They love the smell of coffee and the warm mug. The hit of caffeine wakes them up, which feels good and gets them going for the day. Stepping away from their desk in the middle of the day to get a coffee feels like a much needed break. They love chatting with a friend over coffee. In many ways, coffee has become like wine or smoking, in that people enjoy the social side of it as much as the addictive hit it provides. People make all these associations with coffee: more energy, great taste, delicious smell, catching up with a friend, or having a break from work, but you can enjoy all of those things without the help of a great big latte. Limit yourself to two cups of good-quality coffee or tea a day and keep it clean—by that I mean don't add anything else! If your day revolves around caffeine and sugar then you are causing disruptions to your blood sugar and your energy, weight and appetite will start to suffer. So try caffeine and sugar-free herbal alternatives (more on these in Chapter Two). If you can have one or two cups without any real issue then carry on. As I said before, you know yourself better than anybody.

Finally . . . listen to your gut.

When it comes to deciding what to give up, your gut is one of the best indicators. It's a great communicator known as the second brain. It can really guide us as to what we thrive on and what makes us under par. If you eat bread and bloat or dairy makes you gassy, there's your answer. Your gut is already telling you what you need to give up so listen to it! And don't ignore it. Our digestive system is the foundation of our health and with my clients it is always the first place I check is working well when they come to see me.

CHAPTER 1 · IN A NUTSHELL

Work out your diet weak spot and give it up. Once you have successfully managed that, give up something else.

Eat. Nourish. Glow.

What needs to go / Restocking the fridge / Restocking the pantry / Guide to gluten / Why your kitchen is the heart of your home / Your "What do I do with it?!" guide / How the environment affects your food choices / How to shop smarter / Your toolkit / Cook your way to better health / Detox your desk

The kitchen detox.

—No. 2

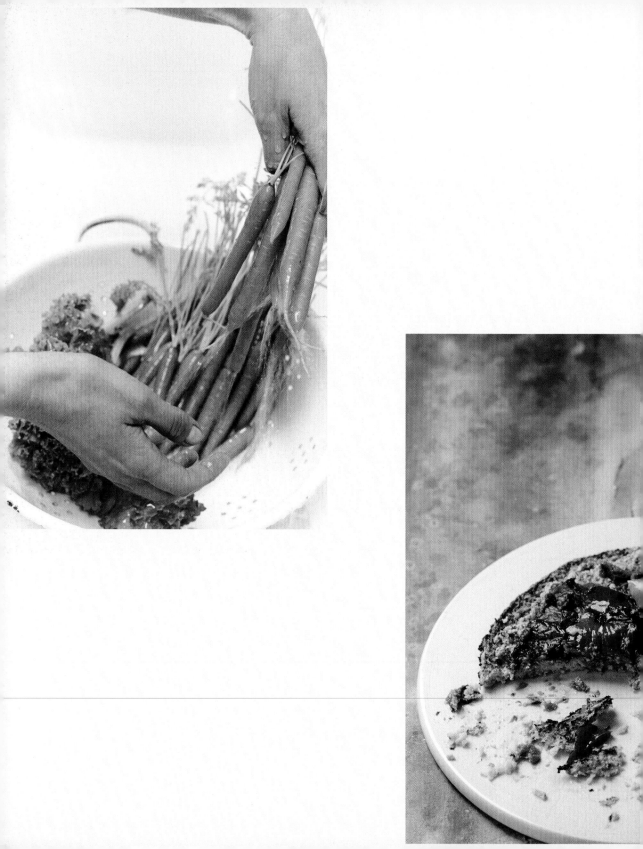

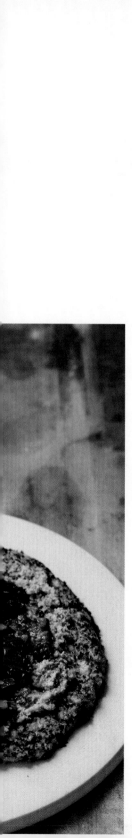

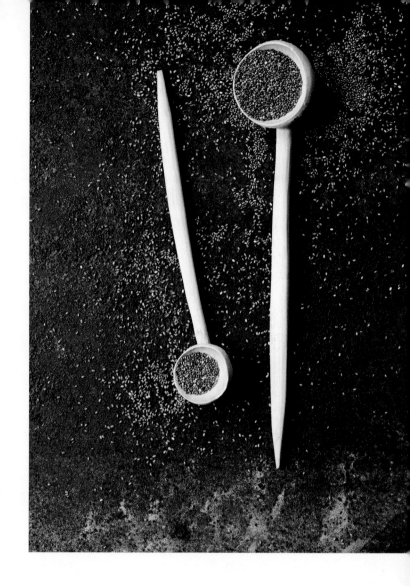

> "You don't have to cook fancy or complicated masterpieces. Just good food from fresh ingredients."

Julia Child, chef

When my new clients start coming to see me, I often begin by discussing the state of their kitchens. Sometimes I actually visit them in person, as a disorganized, junk-filled kitchen leads the very best intentions going astray, so it's essential to prepare your kitchen for success. If you have had a bad day and get home feeling tired and hungry and open the fridge to convenience, nutrient-lacking food, then it will be pretty hard to avoid eating it. I have heard all the excuses in every shape and size. "I got home from work at 8 p.m. and there was nothing in the fridge so I ordered takeout"; "I'd had a stressful day and I ended up eating a whole pack of cookies in front of the TV" or "I couldn't be bothered to cook so I just had pasta again." With my kitchen detox, these scenarios just won't happen.

Let's get the foundations right and get rid of the junk and become organized to allow for a smoother transition as you build on your ONE thing to change over time.

Now, I'm very strict that you throw ALL the junk away—not keep a few in case of emergencies or worry about the waste. Yes, it's wasteful to throw food away but you are not a human trash can, so fill your can with this junk and not your body. Make a decision about what's more important—wasting food or wasting your health. If you have these foods in the house you will eat them at some point, usually when you are tired or stressed. Once you have completed my kitchen detox you won't waste food again because everything you will buy you will use.

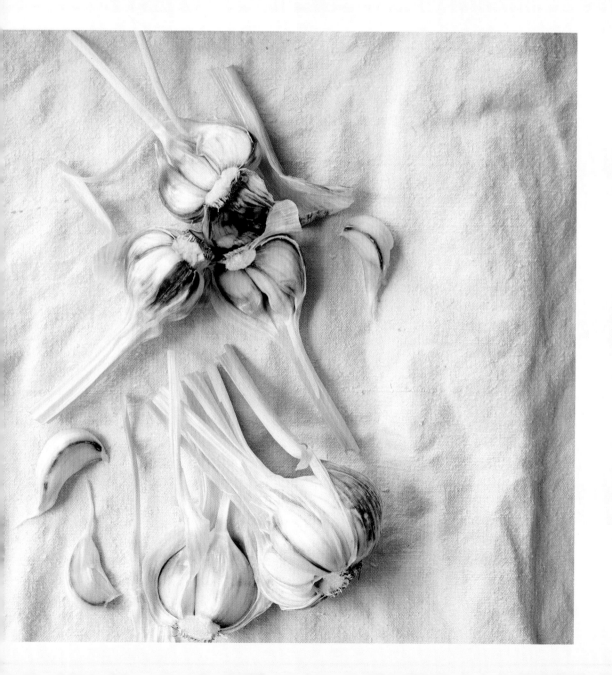

"Don't dig your grave with your own knife and fork."

Old English proverb

Here's what needs to go:

Breakfast cereals These are processed packages of sugar and preservatives with added-in nutrients because they are so lacking in nutrients, the manufacturers need to add some. The packages will have lots of misleading pictures and promises on the front to entice you or your family into wanting to eat them. These kinds of foods set you off on an energy-, sugar-craving rollercoaster that goes on all day long if you start your day this way. If you find that you get energy dips mid-afternoon or lack concentration mid-morning and need to eat something then this is caused by the sugar rollercoaster and it will lead you to believe that you are greedy or lacking willpower. You're not. It's simply your body reacting to the sugar. Don't make life even harder for yourself by having a sugary breakfast. A bowl of cereal is just a bowl of sugary nothingness and it's the worst way to start your day. Throw them out!

🍲 My super-easy healthy cereal

Mix 2 tablespoons chia seeds, 2 tablespoons hemp seeds, a couple of handfuls of mixed nuts chopped, 1 tablespoon sunflower seeds and 1 tablespoon pumpkin seeds together. Add 1 teaspoon ground cinnamon, 1 teaspoon vanilla extract and 1 tablespoon coconut crystals, then add a portion of fresh fruit, such as a handful of fresh raspberries or blueberries and serve with coconut milk or a dollop of coconut yogurt.

Processed and convenience foods Similar to cereals, I call these "Packages and Promises." They are designed to look healthy and flatter your busy life and lack of time to cook for yourself. In reality they are rubbish that will leave you feeling rubbish. As the name suggests, they are heavily processed and no longer resemble their original natural state and no longer contain any nutrients. Most likely they contain a long list of chemicals and they leave your body crying out for nutrients. Once your taste buds get used to these kinds of foods, you crave them more and more. It's not that you are being greedy and lazy it's the food doing that to you, so throw out all your cans, ready-made meals and everything else that comes in a package and has a long ingredients list. By the end of this book I want you to be buying ingredients, not meals!

Margarine Yuck! Since it became popular, just after World War II, margarine has claimed to be a healthy version of butter—oh what a foul deception this is. Butter is such a pure product and one I have always encouraged clients to eat (if they are OK to eat dairy) rather than a tub of dyed yellow plastic chemicals with healthy pictures and words on the front. "Packages and Promises!" No, butter isn't fattening and, yes, it does contain fat, but these fats are essential for our well-being. OK don't eat a stick of butter a day but it's a fine product to use if you aren't sensitive to dairy products. If you wish to eat butter, my advice is to ensure it's organic (which means not filled with chemicals and hormones) and grass-fed (which means produced from cattle that have been humanely raised and eat the food they were meant to eat) that way it's in the most natural form possible. Keep your foods pure and as close to their natural state as possible. Let's not let our kitchens and health be highjacked.

Canned meals I'm referring to foods covered in sauces that are heated and ready to eat such as soups or SpaghettiOs here. Canning foods isn't a very healthy way to store food, but I'm not going to say that you won't find the odd can of tomatoes, coconut milk or chickpeas in my cupboard, as you will; they can be useful staples, but keep them to a minimum. Studies show that small amounts of chemicals and toxins from the can leach into the food, so they are not something we want to use daily. In addition, the food in cans has often been prepared in a way that makes it last longer, which severely reduces its nutrient value, as well as many having added sugar, refined salt and preservatives to keep it from going bad, so read the labels and choose the ones that only contain water.

Gluten grains In Chapter One I discussed the negative way gluten grains impact our health, so they have to go in my kitchen detox.

Salad dressings Most store-bought salad dressings contain sugar and some contain gluten. They are a sickly, sugary way of trying to add flavor to your salad; add natural flavors instead (see page 76 for my dressing recipe).

Biscuits, cakes and sweets If you don't have these types of food in your house you won't be able to eat them in a comatose state at the end of a long day or when you are bored and looking for a distraction. Don't hold on to a few as a safety net—throw them all out! Just because they are sold on the shelves does not mean that they are safe to eat. They are not. For you or anyone else in your household. If you buy them, they will get eaten and the cascade of sugar cravings and hunger kicks in. They are easier to kick than you think, but you have to start by just not buying them—for anyone. This goes for the "healthy, organic, gluten-free" ones too.

Yogurts We have been grossly misled to believe that yogurts are a healthy product. While they do contain protein, probiotics and calcium and are advertised to support gut health, if you dig a little deeper, they are in fact a bit of a cheat. The probiotic content is minimal so it's better to take a good-quality probiotic capsule instead. The calcium content isn't enough on its own as calcium needs magnesium and vitamin D to be utilized for bone density. Dark leafy green vegetables and nuts are a far better choice. Yes, yogurts do contain protein but so do many other great foods, such as eggs, nuts and seeds. Most alarming of all are the "healthy, low-fat" varieties, which sadly contain the equivalent amount of sugar to a can of fizzy drink. I discussed dairy and the concerns for some in Chapter One so I won't go on here, but it's now time to let go of the low-fat, high sugar products that are just not what they say they are.

Table or cooking salt This is actually a processed form of salt that is not recognized by our bodies and contains chemicals. Table salt contains additives to make it free-flowing. Ferrocyanide, talc and silica aluminate are just some of the chemicals added. It lacks the essential trace minerals, which are the components of real salt that we need to survive. It can disrupt the body's fluid balance, which can lead to cellulite and more serious conditions, such as arthritis, gout and kidney problems. Sometimes it has aluminum added to it, which is linked to Alzheimer's. Eating lots of restaurant or processed food, both of which can have large quantities of this unnatural salt can be detrimental to our health. You don't need it at home—buy sea salt or Himalayan pink salt (see page 56) instead.

Anything out of date It sounds obvious, but most of us have food that's out of date in our kitchens, especially tucked away at the back of our cupboards, including out of date spices. Throw them all out—it's time to start fresh and get organized so you can see what you have and what you need.

That's the elimination process. Now for the restock. Let's start with the fridge.

Protein Allocate one shelf of your fridge to be dedicated to protein because each of your meals should contain it, for example fish, meat or chicken.

Non-meat protein such as cooked legumes, nuts and seeds.

Salad and vegetables Every single one of your meals should contain vegetables. Buy anything and everything you fancy and swap it around week by week so you are getting a good mix. Organic and in season is best, and as a general rule try to eat the most colorful vegetables you can find—aim for the rainbow. We all know greens are great—we have been told that for years, and they are great so keep eating them, but don't forget other colors, too. The colors in vegetables are a health powerhouse of phytonutrients that help reduce the risk of heart disease, cancer and diabetes, so when you are shopping for vegetables picture a rainbow and try to buy as many colorful ones as possible—red peppers and tomatoes, orange sweet potatoes, carrots and squash, purple sprouting broccoli, yellow sweet corn, deep purple blackberries and blueberries.

Your favorite dairy alternative like coconut milk or a nut milk and coconut yogurts, and feta or goat's cheese if you eat those.

54

Then for the pantry.

Healthy flavors Fresh, dried (or frozen) herbs, black pepper, sea salt, lemons, chilies and garlic are brilliant for throwing into recipes to add healthy flavors.

Olive oil and coconut oil Olive oil is great for drizzling over salads and already-roasted vegetables but don't cook with it. It has a very low tolerance for heat, and burning food with it is negating the benefits. Over the years we have been encouraged to use olive oil rather than sunflower or vegetable oil, and rightly so because it's a healthier option, and the others can't be heated either. So just use olive oil cold for added flavor and cook with coconut oil, butter, ghee or avocado oil, all which have a higher tolerance for heat.

Glass jars of legumes, like chickpeas and lentils Avoid cans as much as possible. If you do use them, make sure they don't have added sugar or preservatives in them.

Coconut flour, rice flour and gram (chickpea) flour These gluten-free flours are my staples for baking or thickening foods like sauces.

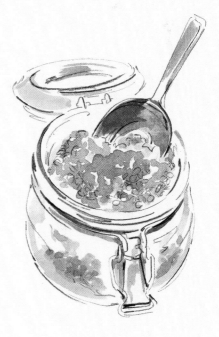

Brown rice, pasta or noodles or rice paper wraps These can be great for occasional treats and certainly if you are trying to wean your household off gluten-containing products. They are still a form of sugar to your body so use occasionally, not daily.

Quinoa This is a useful seed, not grain, that can be a good alternative to rice or couscous. It can cause digestive issues for some people and it's not something I eat often, but I do have it for odd occasions. It's naturally gluten-free and a rich source of protein so it's good for vegans and vegetarians.

Himalayan pink sea salt crystals The most natural form of salt available with the highest mineral content.

Good-quality coffee If you have the caffeine habit, then invest in good-quality, organic coffee. As I discussed in Chapter One, I encourage you to keep it to a maximum of two cups per day and avoid adding anything to it. Good-quality coffee has a great flavor so you don't need to make it frothy and add sugar. As caffeine can disrupt sleep for some, make sure you drink it before midday.

Apple cider vinegar This is an excellent vinegar to use in salad dressings or to drink in warm water. It is hypothesized to help burn fat and aid digestion among many other things.

Simple salad dressing

Mix some apple cider vinegar with a little olive oil, mustard powder, fresh rosemary, garlic and a pinch of sea salt and freshly ground black pepper to make a lovely salad dressing. I also use this mix to marinate vegetables, fish or chicken.

Turmeric: This spice is more of a medicine in my mind, and well known for its role in reducing inflammation. I try to encourage my clients to include turmeric in their diets where they can, for example in curries, soups, dressings and shakes (See my Anti-inflammatory Dressing recipe on page 76).

🥣 Turmeric tea

Boil some water, add some fresh turmeric, fresh ginger and a slice or two of lemon.

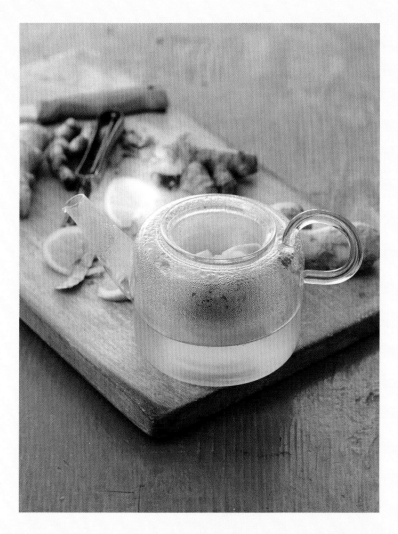

"You can eat all the junk food you want. As long as you make it all from scratch."

COELIAC U.K.

Guide to gluten

Not gluten-free

Barley—including products that contain malted barley, such as malt drinks, beer, ales, lager and stouts

Bulgur wheat—partially-cooked wheat

Couscous—granules made from semolina

Durum wheat—wheat used in making pasta and bread

Einkorn—ancient form of wheat

Emmer—wheat, also know as farro

Kamut—ancient wheat grain

Pearl barley—barley that has the hull and bran removed

Rye—closely related to barley and wheat

Semolina—coarse particles of wheat, used to make pasta and desserts

Spelt—ancient form of wheat

Triticale—a cross between wheat and rye

Wheat—used to make bread, pasta, cookies and cake

May contain gluten—need to check by reading labels carefully

Barley malt extract—used as a flavoring. Some breakfast cereals containing barley malt extract are suitable

Oats—often contaminated with gluten, but most people can eat contaminated oats

Gluten-free

Agar agar—from algae, can be used as an alternative to gelatin

Almond—often ground and used as an alternative to flour in baking

Amaranth—traditional plant used in Africa

Buckwheat—used to make flour and noodles

Carageenan—from red seaweed, used as a food additive

Cassava (manioc)—the white or yellow flesh can be boiled and used as an accompaniment for meat dishes. Tapioca starch is produced from dried cassava root

Chestnut—ground and used in flour

Corn—also called maize, used for flour

Flaxseeds (linseeds)—seeds can be added to muesli

Gram flour (besan)—from ground chickpeas

Hemp—flour and seeds used in bakery and cereal products

Hops—used in the brewing of beer

Maize—also called corn, used for flour

Millet/bajra—cereal used in porridge

Mustard—plant used for flour and powder

Polenta—cooked cornmeal

Potato—used to thicken sauces and soups, flour/starch used in baking

Legumes (peas, beans, lentils)—can be ground into flour and used in a variety of dishes

Quinoa—closely related to beets and spinach, used in muesli, salads and baking

Rice—for example wild, arborio, basmati

Sago—starch extracted from sago palms, used as a thickener

Sesame—seeds used in baking

Sorghum—sorghum malt used in gluten-free brewing

Soy—bean ground to make soy flour

Tapioca—starch from the root of the cassava, commonly used to make tapioca pudding

Teff—a grass with small seeds, used to make flour

Urd/urid/urad flour—ground lentils

Why your kitchen should be the heart of your home

Many of us—especially those living far away from their families in big cities, or who are busy with work—have lost the art of preparing nourishing meals and sitting down alone or with loved ones to enjoy them. I live alone and I still take the time to cook a proper meal for myself. In fact, doing so is often the most relaxing part of my day. Whether I'm on my own or with friends or my family, I love the process of creating a meal from start to finish. Everyone can get involved, including children who will love whisking eggs or counting out ingredients, so I really encourage that we get back to cooking our way to better happiness and health. Give it a try if you aren't already.

Your "What do I do with it?!" guide

Most people interested in healthy eating know that foods like chia seeds are good for them. They might even know what they look or taste like, but I have found that many of us just don't know what to do with them. Here are a few tips on what to do with some of the healthy foods you have been hearing about or may have bought but just don't quite know what to do with!

Chia seeds

What are they? A unique and nutritionally complex seed from a flowering plant in the mint family, chia seeds come from central and southern Mexico and Guatemala.

Why are they so good? They are rich in omega-3 essential fats, protein and antioxidants. They are also very filling and a great source of fiber.

What do I do with them? Soak them in your liquid of choice—they taste best with a creamy liquid such as nut milk, which causes them to swell up and resemble frogs' eggs, then add fruit, ground cinnamon or vanilla and they make a delicious and healthy breakfast, dessert, yogurt or oatmeal replacement. You can also become more creative by using different ingredients, such as raw chocolate and other spices. They are very versatile . . .

Coconut oil

What is it? The oil obtained from the flesh of a coconut.

Why is it so good? It's a healthy source of saturated fat, which is beneficial for helping with weight loss. It also contains lauric acid, which has antimicrobial and antibacterial properties.

What do I do with it? Use coconut oil to cook with instead of olive oil (it has a higher tolerance for heat than olive oil). Use the extra virgin oil for curries or Thai dishes as it has a coconut flavor, and use the "no aroma" butter for more traditional or Mediterranean flavored dishes that won't work so well with the coconutty flavor. It can be blended into smoothies, used in healthy desserts and to "cream" coffee or tea. It also can be used on skin and hair, as a sun cream and for stretch marks.

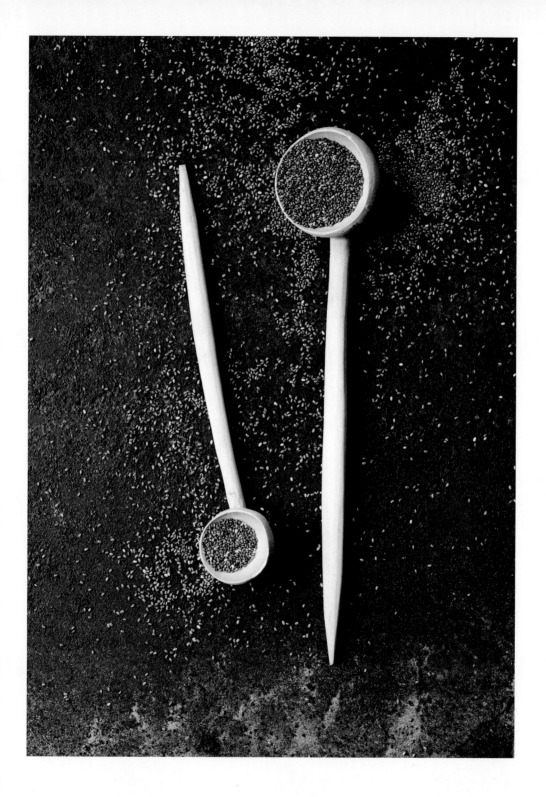

Himalayan pink salt

What is it? One of the purest forms of salt on earth.
Why is it so good? Unlike refined table or cooking salt, Himalayan pink salt is rich in vitamins and minerals and free from toxins. It is reported to have many benefits from improving sleep, reducing muscle cramps, regulating water content throughout the body and supporting respiratory health. This is the best salt to buy and cook with.
What do I do with it? Simply use instead of regular salt to flavor food or to bathe in.

Apple cider vinegar

What is it? A type of vinegar made from apples.
Why is it so good? It's great for detoxing, helps balance blood sugar levels and reduces blood pressure. It can also help to reduce body fat especially around the midsection.
What do I do with it? Mix it with olive oil and mustard powder to make a salad dressing. Add it to soups or stews for flavor. You can also add it to hot water and drink to aid digestion.

Legumes

What are they? Lentils and beans.
Why are they so good? They are a rich source of iron, potassium, magnesium and zinc and a great source of fiber. They do contain protein and so are a key staple for vegans and vegetarians, however, they are also a carbohydrate so I don't recommend my clients eating them in large quantities or too frequently. They don't agree with everyone so this is a personal choice to eat them or not.
What do I do with them? Legumes are great in curries, soups, stews, burgers and salads.

How your environment affects your food choices

Several studies from Cornell University in the U.S. have found that the way our kitchen is organized affects our food choices. If you have a messy fridge with sugary or convenience foods at eye level, you will make bad choices. If you have a well-organized and well-stocked fridge full of healthy options (see page 54), you will make better choices.

How to shop smarter

Food manufacturers and supermarkets have been highjacking our food choices for years. There's a reason why you pop into a supermarket to buy two things and come out with twenty. There's also a reason why you can't just eat a small handful of chips in a bag. Supermarkets are designed by very clever people who want you to spend more money, so they arrange their aisles and displays in such a way to seduce you to want more. Every single supermarket layout decision, from the lighting to where food is displayed, is geared toward getting you to spend more money—usually on processed foods.

Food manufacturers also employ a tactic to make you want to eat more of their product. With promises on the packaging and a cocktail of processed salt, sugar and additives in the ingredients they lure us into a false sense of security and quite frankly have stolen our taste buds and our connection with our food choices. Don't be highjacked by their tricks! Avoid "Packages and Promises" and just eat real food.

It wasn't always this way. We used to buy fresh food every few days from local shops like the butchers and corner grocers. Food went bad quickly because it came from a local source and it didn't contain preservatives. We didn't have shelves crammed with cookbooks. Instead we were taught to cook by our mothers, aunts or grandmothers and were very confident in our ability to cook a family meal from scratch— we had no other choice. Food manufacturers have completely insulted our cooking confidence. They have come between us and the kitchen all under the guise of making our life easier and more convenient, and flattering our sense of busyness. Why bother making proper gravy when

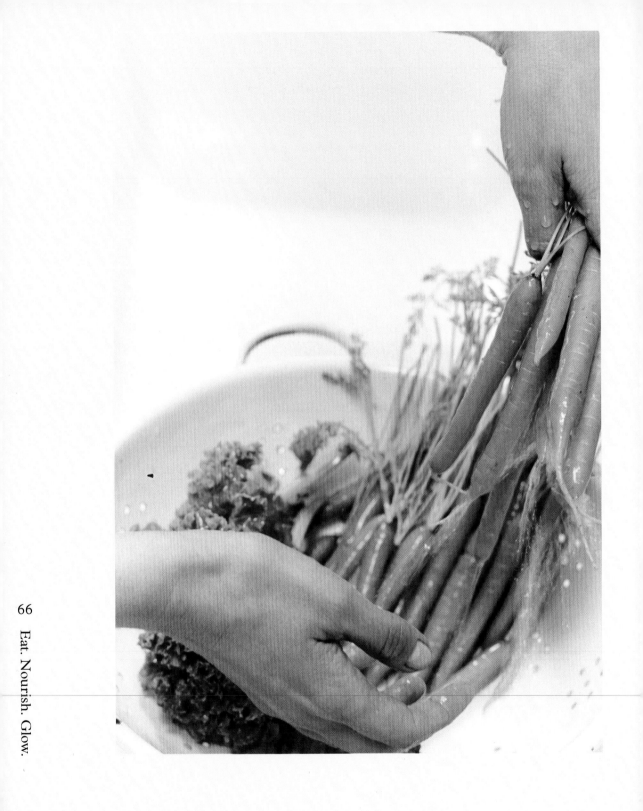

Eat. Nourish. Glow.

you add boiling water to granules? Why bother making a curry sauce from scratch when you can just buy a jar? Why make a meal when you can just pierce a film of plastic wrap and put a ready-made one in the microwave?

Being busy is the new status symbol—it means we are important, good at our jobs and valued by others. The food industry has tapped into our feelings of self-worth by giving us the message, "You're too busy to cook yourself a meal so here we've done it for you." We have fallen for their tricks and our health has paid the price. They have corrupted our food choices too by filling convenience food with so much sugar, sweeteners and additives that our taste buds start to think that this is normal and forget how delicious good-quality home-cooked food tastes. My clients salivate over my food simply because they have been eating bland, artificially sweetened, beige and "dead" food for so long.

If you break the convenience habit and start making meals from scratch—which takes no time at all when you know how—you will never look back. Food from scratch is the single most important thing you can do for your health, and it's so easy. When I show clients how to throw together a spicy Thai sauce or a soup from raw ingredients they are always surprised at how quick and simple it is—but only if you have the ingredients in the first place!

When it comes to shopping I tell my clients to keep things simple. If it's got a barcode or a "promise," don't buy it. Healthy, real, whole food doesn't need to sell itself. Avocados don't have "heart healthy" on the package, do they? An organic steak doesn't make any grand promise about being a fantastic source of iron, does it? So if your food is trying to sell itself, don't buy it. If it has a long list of ingredients, don't buy it. Freshly made pesto, which has around three or four ingredients, is fine. A stir-fry sauce containing 20 different ingredients isn't. Buy your own fresh ingredients and assemble them yourself. Don't let your health and your common sense be taken hostage by convenience food.

"What I have learned is this; we have to cook our way out of this mess."

Dr. Mark Hyman M.D.

My ditch and switch guide to shopping

Ditch	Switch	Need to know
Cow's milk	Coconut milk, unsweetened almond, cashew or rice milk	Although dairy has many positive attributes, there is increasing evidence that it may be best avoided or at least kept to a minimum. It is one of the seven most allergenic foods and can trigger both digestive and systemic health problems such as eczema, asthma, increased mucus production and low mood. 95% of the world's population (individuals not of northern European ethnicity) are lactose intolerant, which contributes to digestive issues such as diarrhea and flatulence. Contrary to the myth created by the dairy

industry, dairy is not required for bone health—nuts, seeds, legumes, small fish and greens, such as broccoli, provide better, more absorbable sources of calcium than dairy. Dairy consumption is linked to an increased risk of hormone-related cancers as it contains a growth hormone called IGF-1 (insulin-like growth factor), which is great for young, growing calves but not so good for the human breast, ovaries or prostate. Dairy is a source of animal fat, which can have a pro-inflammatory effect due to its high levels of arachidonic acid. Finally, the dairy industry is not great for animal welfare, the environment or sustainability. If you decide to eat dairy, choose organic and if possible, find a raw dairy producer—many can deliver around the U.K.

| Pre-made salad dressings | Olive oil, lemon juice, sea salt and freshly ground pepper. Add fresh mustard powder, apple cider vinegar and fresh herbs for a French-style dressing | Instead of using olive oil, pre-made salad dressings often use cheaper vegetable oils that are high in omega-6. This affects our omega-3 to 6 ratio and can lead to increased inflammation. Many pre-made dressings contain high amounts of sugar and salt. Artificial preservatives may also be used. |
| Sodas | Fizzy coconut water, sparkling | A standard 12-ounce soft drink contains between 4–7 teaspoons of |

water with fresh lime, lemon or orange squeezed in, fresh mint or rosemary, fruit or herb ice cubes, kombucha, iced herbal teas

Note Fruit juice is high in sugar so if you are using it, dilute it 50:50 with water/ sparkling water.

sugar, which will quickly enter the bloodstream leading to an insulin spike. High fructose corn syrup (HFCS) is sometimes the sugar used in fizzy drinks (more so in the U.S.), which not only impacts calories but also contributes to fatty liver disease and elevated cholesterol levels even more heavily than regular sugar or glucose. "Lite" or sugar-free soft drinks usually replace sugar with sweeteners, which are artificial chemicals that are an unnecessary burden on the body. Research has shown that low-cal drinks do not appear to help with weight loss.

| Ice cream | Coconut ice cream or frozen homemade smoothies | See dairy, above. Sugar in all forms is best avoided—but if you want a frozen treat, consider dairy-free alternatives with lowest sugar content. |

| Milk chocolate | 70% dark chocolate or sugar-free, raw chocolates available from health food stores. For the more adventurous, make your own with cacao | See dairy above. Chocolate is often cited as a superfood as it is rich in antioxidants and minerals. However, this applies more specifically to raw chocolate. Processed chocolate is a little less super, but good-quality dark chocolate with over 70% cocoa is better than milk chocolate. Did you know that the word "cacao" describes raw chocolate, while "cocoa" describes processed |

	powder, coconut butter and coconut crystals	chocolate? Go for cacao where you can! Milk chocolate is lower in cocoa and high in sugar, canceling out much of what is "super" about this "food of the gods."
Wheat flour	Brown rice flour, coconut flour, chickpea flour, amaranth flour	Modern wheat, as we know it, has been bred over the years into a grain which is vastly different from the wheat first farmed in Mesopotamia. Gluten levels are much higher in modern wheat, which is probably a major contributor to the surge in gluten sensitivities and celiac disease over the last 50 years. Gluten has been shown to irritate the gut lining, potentially leading to intestinal permeability. Even for those who are not wheat sensitive, it is best to try and diversify your sources of carbohydrate so that you aren't eating a "monochrome" diet of wheat with bread, pasta and baked goods for every meal.
Sugar	Coconut crystals, stevia, xylitol, maple syrup or honey	The best way to approach sugar reduction is to accept that the less sugar you eat, the faster your taste buds will adapt and the quicker your cravings will go—I promise, just hang in there! The less-processed, natural sugars, such as maple syrup or honey, are somewhat better than white table sugar, but it is still sugar and will still trigger an insulin response.

Coconut nectar and granulated coconut sugar are dehydrated nectar or saps from palm trees—both, especially the latter, are significantly more nutritious (and tasty) than most other sugars and are a better option, but still should be used in moderation.

Natural low-calorie sweeteners such as stevia or xylitol can help to bridge the gap but ultimately, the less you depend on sugar or sweeteners, the faster you will adapt to low sugar eating habits.

| Margarine | Organic butter, ghee or coconut butter | Margarine is usually made from oils, which contain the more pro-inflammatory omega-6s. Historically, they were higher in trans fats and although this has improved somewhat, I still believe that we are better off eating foods that have not been heavily manipulated. Butter has had a bad rap for many years but I would recommend it (in moderation) over margarine for those who are not dairy sensitive. Clarified butter may be better tolerated for those that are. Butter is a great source of butyric acid, which actually helps to heal the gut. Coconut oil/fat is a great butter alternative and it can spread well at room temperature. If you don't want the coconut flavor, try one of the brands that are "aroma free." Coconut oil is also well suited for cooking at high temperatures as the oils are very stable and don't oxidize easily. |

Bread	Buckwheat or millet bread, Genius bread, rice bread, quinoa bread, chickpea flatbread	This book will introduce new ways to include carbohydrates into your diet without depending on bread. However, there are certain meals that just don't feel complete without some kind of bread as a vehicle. Try out the various alternatives to find which ones work well for you. It is possible to store many of these in the freezer so you can just take what you need each day. Note: Many gluten-free breads improve with toasting.
Crackers	Flax or other seed crackers	Try the many different types of gluten-free crackers that are now available online or in health food stores, but check the ingredients as they are not all healthy. I suggest sticking to raw varieties, or making your own.
Pizza	Buckwheat pizza dough, chickpea flatbread, vegetable bases such as cauliflower, zucchini or eggplant	Vegetable pizza doughs are surprisingly good! Or else you can use a gluten-free flatbread or pre-made pizza dough so you can create a pizza treat.
Chips	Sweet potato chips	Sweet potato has a much lower GI (glycemic index) than white potatoes while also being more nutritious and tasty. It also lends itself to many different flavors so get creative.

Grains	Quinoa, gluten-free oats, brown rice, wild rice, buckwheat	Using gluten-free grains helps to break the habit of depending too heavily on wheat-based carbs all the time.
Crisps	Kale chips, homemade vegetable chips	Most of us love the texture of a chip. Thankfully healthier versions can fill that gap. Kale chips or root vegetable chips are a great healthier alternative and easy to make yourself using coconut oil, herbs and sea salt.
Bottled sauces	Fresh, dried or frozen herbs, sea salt and freshly ground black pepper, garlic, chilies, lemongrass, lemon and lime	Most pre-made sauces are high in sugar and salt. Try making your own salsas or marinades using fresh ingredients. You will soon find that they taste better while also being great for your health.
Yogurt	Coconut yogurt or soaked blended nuts mixed with fruit or natural sweetness	See dairy above. Coconut yogurt is a great alternative, which can be used in sweet or savory dishes, as a replacement for yogurt, sour cream, crème fraîche and cream. When going dairy free, a little creamy treat is always great.
Coffee & tea	Green tea, rooibos, chai	Coffee and tea aren't bad; they just aren't great if consumed in excess or used to replace meals: 1–2 black teas or coffees total per day is fine in my book. However, if you find that caffeine gives you palpitations, you

may be better going for herbal teas instead. Many people find that after the initial adjustment of removing caffeine completely from their diet, they have more energy throughout the day.

Mayonnaise	Tahini, raw nut butters	Homemade mayonnaise with olive oil is fine in moderation. However, most store-bought mayonnaises will be made from cheaper oils, higher in omega-6. You can substitute tahini or nut butters in many recipes or sauces that call for mayonnaise.
Soy sauce	Coconut aminos, tamari	Soy contains gluten so isn't ideal for following a gluten-free diet. Try coconut aminos (the sap of the coconut tree), or tamari (GF soy sauce) instead.
Beer, rum, sweet cocktails and sugary mixers	Vodka, gin, red wine, mixers such as sparkling water, fresh citrus juice, naturally light tonic water	I am partial to the occasional tipple but always try to go for options that are lower in sugar, such as white spirits with soda and lime or tonic. Some red wines can be high in sugar but at least they may also supply antioxidants. Order a bottle of water for the table and try to remember to drink it alongside the alcohol!

Homemade harissa

½ cup dried chilies
1 tsp caraway seeds
1 tsp coriander seeds
1 tsp cumin seeds
3–4 garlic cloves, peeled
1 tsp sea salt
2 tbsp extra virgin olive oil

Place the chilies in a heatproof bowl, cover with boiling water and leave to stand for 30 minutes.

Meanwhile, toast all the spices in a dry frying pan over a low-medium heat, shaking or stirring occasionally to prevent them from burning. When the spices are fragrant, remove them from the pan and grind them in a mortar and pestle.

Drain the chilies, remove the stems and seeds, then combine the chilies with the ground spices, garlic and salt.

Put the mixture in a food processor and while the processor is running, slowly drizzle in the olive oil and process to form a smooth and thick paste. Taste and adjust seasonings.

Anti-inflammatory dressing

½ avocado
Juice and zest of 1 orange
2 tbsp apple cider vinegar
1-inch piece fresh tumeric root or 3 tsp ground tumeric
1 clove garlic, peeled.
¾-inch cube of fresh ginger, peeled
1 teaspoon coconut crystals or raw honey if you need it sweeter
A splash of olive oil
Filtered water, as needed
Sea salt and freshly ground pepper

Place all ingredients in a blender and blend until smooth.
Store in a glass jar in the fridge—it will last for up to one week.

Your toolkit

Getting going in the kitchen is so much harder without the right tools. I sometimes can't cook in other people's kitchens as a different pan can change a whole dish, as can unfamiliar ingredients. It's not about buying snazzy and designer items, but there are some staples that will certainly help you enjoy your time in the kitchen. See page 260 for suppliers.

Knives

One of the most important cooking tools in your kitchen are your knives. Every kitchen should have at least one very sharp good-quality knife. Well-sharpened knives are a pleasure to use and I get my own knives sharpened twice a year. I'm amazed by the number of clients who have bad knives that don't slice through lean protein and vegetables properly making prepping food so much harder and more of a hassle—it would discourage me from cooking. When you start to prepare food with a properly sharpened knife you will see how much easier it is.

Tongs

These are awesome and have lots of uses—flipping burgers, tossing salads, sautéing vegetables, blanching vegetable or rice noodles, use with griddle pans and steaming greens—they are a must for quick and nifty cooks.

Vitamix blender

This blender is a serious bit of kit and pretty much a must for health food lovers. It's pricy but it repays you—it's a cherished part of my kitchen and used daily. Why it's so superior to regular blenders is its extra tough and high speed blades that can turn virtually anything into a liquid—yes even an avocado pit can be liquidized! It's great for making nut milks, vegetable smoothies, soups, sauces, ice creams or sorbets and nut creams—oh yes, and I blend my coffee and coconut oil this way. If you can't afford a Vitamix then go for NutriBullet instead.

Cold press juicer

This is a juicer that doesn't use heat to extract the goodness from the fruit and vegetables, therefore providing a higher nutrient juice . . . now that can't be bad.

Hand-held blender

This is great for making pestos, dressings, sauces, blending soups or puréeing vegetables, such as peas, parsnips or sweet potatoes. Every kitchen needs one.

Microplane

A nifty and easier to use grater—excellent for sprinkling a little bit of citrus zest over a dish or for finely grating ginger, garlic, chilies, lemongrass or nutmeg. I use mine every day.

Spiralizer

Another favorite! I use it to make carrot ribbons to add to raw salads or zucchini or squash spaghetti. Here's a quick recipe.

Vegetable spaghetti

Boil a pan of water, then pour into a heatproof bowl and add a little salt. Using carrot, butternut squash or zucchini, make your "spaghetti" noodles and place in the bowl of hot water for 2 minutes. Drain and rinse under cold running water then stir in some pesto, olive oil and fresh lemon zest. A tiny grating of truffle is amazing if you have some.

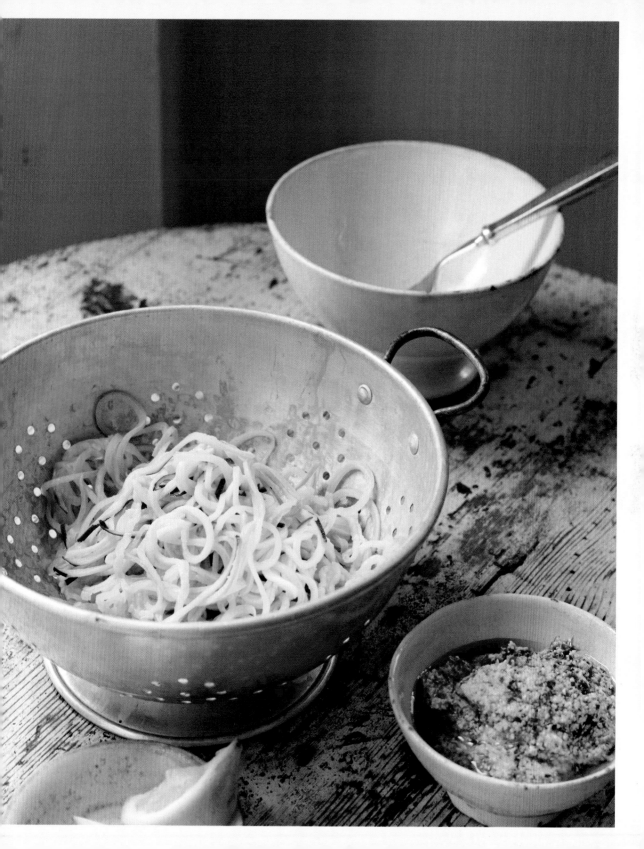

Zucchini spaghetti with a choice of sauces

Use a spiralizer to make the zucchini spirals as explained on page 78 in the Vegetable spaghetti recipe. Then choose your favorite topping from the suggestions below:

🥣 Creamy Thai sauce

½ cup cashew nuts
1 red chili
Juice of 1 lime
½-inch cube of fresh ginger, peeled
1 garlic clove, peeled
Coconut oil
Fresh cilantro, for sprinkling

Soak the cashews in a bowl of water for 2–3 minutes, then drain and put in a blender with the remaining ingredients, except the cilantro. Blend until creamy, adding water, if necessary. Pour the sauce over the "zucchetti" and sprinkle fresh cilantro over the top. Serve with shrimp and red or yellow peppers.

🥣 Herby pesto

½ cup cashews
Juice and zest of 1 lemon
1 garlic clove, peeled
A handful of fresh basil
A handful of fresh parsley
Sea salt and freshly ground black pepper
Olive oil

Soak the cashews in a bowl of water overnight, then drain and put in a blender with the remaining ingredients. Blend, keeping a little bit of texture. Pour the pesto over the "zucchetti."

Lemon juice, lemon zest, olive oil, sea salt and freshly ground black pepper are great on yellow "zucchetti" and served as a side dish with fish or chicken. Or serve it alongside your favorite Bolognese sauce, as mentioned on page 138.

"Zucchetti" can be made with other vegetables, such as sweet potato, carrot, parsnip, squash, beet, and a mix of different types of vegetables together looks wonderful.

They can be served completely raw but I prefer to blanch them in hot water for 2–3 minutes first before eating.

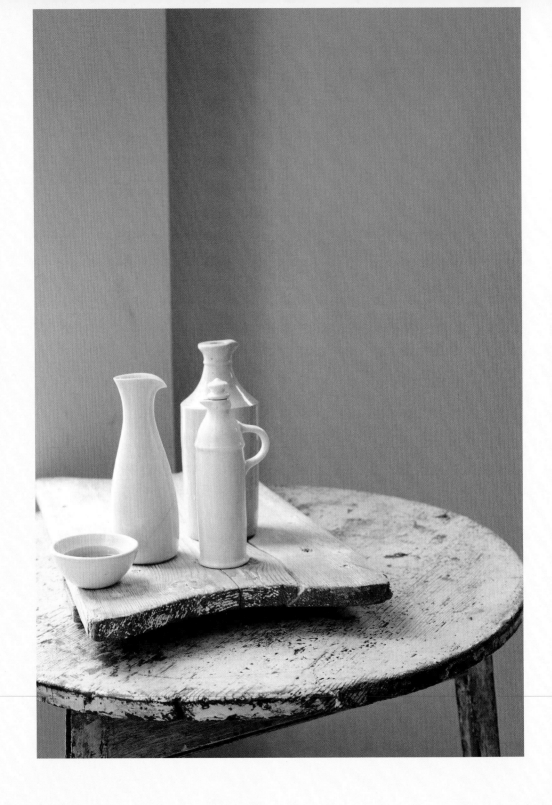

Eat. Nourish. Glow.

A good set of bowls

I use stainless-steel bowls for mixing salads and mixing ground turkey, lamb or beef to make burgers. They are also great for baking mixtures and tossing vegetables in herbs and spices.

Cook your way to better health

Microwaves

I don't have one and I urge my clients to use theirs as little as possible, if at all. Microwaves denature the nutrients in food—and it's the nutrients that we need! The types of foods that require microwaving also tend to be nutritionally empty and processed, like prepared meals, ready-made soups and rice. If you do use a microwave to heat something up—ideally something you have made yourself—then limit the damage by putting it into a china or glass bowl and covering with another china plate. Don't ever heat plastic in the microwave as the process encourages the BPA to be leached from the plastic container into the food.

Poaching

I steam and poach a lot because it's easy and requires little attention or washing up—I am fundamentally quite lazy! Bring a pan of water to a boil and add some flavor like garlic, onions or spices. Then add some meat, poultry or fish, cover with a lid, turn off the heat and let it slowly cook through. It's that simple. Chicken takes around 20 minutes whereas fish takes about 7 minutes. As the meat or fish poaches, it holds onto the moisture and flavor from the water leaving it beautifully succulent and tender. I will always make enough for another meal and store it in the fridge.

Steam-frying

This is a great way to cook flavors like garlic, onion, chilies and
ginger before adding the meat or fish. In a frying pan, add a couple
of tablespoons of water. Let the heat from the water steam them. Keep
sprinkling in small amounts of water whenever it starts to dry out
so keep a jug close by. This is not about boiling the food, just gently
steaming slowly to break down the food leaving it beautifully tender.

Sautéing

This is where you heat coconut oil, butter or ghee in a pan and let the
vegetables "sweat," not burn or blacken, which produces cancer promoting
compounds. This is why olive oil should be kept for cold use, such as salad
dressings or pouring over cooked vegetables. For this reason, I always suggest
that you use coconut oil, butter or ghee (clarified butter) to cook with.

Sous vide

A fantastic way to cook meats perfectly by placing meat and your flavor of
choice into a water bath. My only issue with the sous vide machines is the
plastic bags and as you already know, I try to limit the plastic in my life,
so I source the best quality BPA-free plastic bags to use when cooking with
this method.

Slow cooker

Ideal for making bone broths, soups and stews, this is an essential piece of
equipment for a busy home. Just put everything in the cooker, set it before
you leave in the morning and it's ready for when you get home.

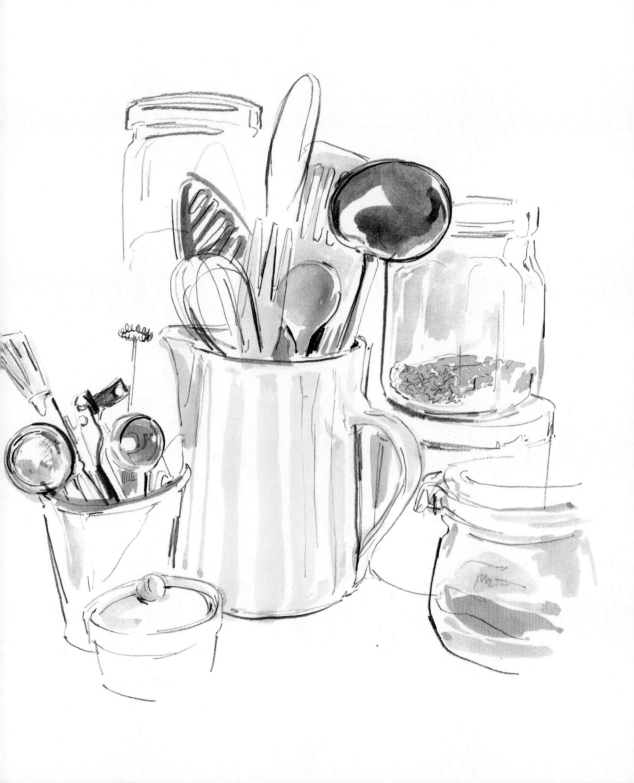

Detox your desk

If you spend a large part of your day at a desk, treat your desk to a mini detox too. Don't keep sugary foods in the drawers—no matter how much you tuck them away out of sight, you will inevitably reach for them the moment you feel stressed or when it's 3 p.m. and you are tired and craving a pick-me-up. Although I'm not a fan of snacking (see Chapter Four) I appreciate that if you have a meeting that runs through lunch, or you are stuck at work past dinnertime, it's important you have healthy snacks on hand to keep you away from the vending machine or local coffee shop. If this is familiar to you then I suggest nuts, seeds, fresh fruit and raw organic seed bars. Don't forget hydration at work—many of my clients admit they go through a whole day without a glass of water. Being dehydrated can often lead us to eat the wrong foods and also make us tired and foggy so we think we need a coffee and a piece of cake to pick us up. Instead, try keeping a big jug of water on your desk and add any (or a mix) of the following to it: a wedge of lemon, lime, orange or cucumber, or some fresh herbs like mint and rosemary. Last, make a bottle of salad dressing with olive oil and apple cider vinegar at the beginning of each month. This will liven up your lunch and keep you away from sugary, artificial flavorings like vinaigrettes and creamy salad dressings that come in prepared store-bought salads.

Throw out all the junk in your kitchen, keep it well stocked with nourishing foods and invest in a few new utensils that will help make cooking healthier and more pleasurable.

What type of eater are you? /
Emotional eater / Disordered
eater / Mindless eater / How to
find your grace around food /
Don't give food a label / Eat
mindfully and consciously /
Make eating a priority / Avoid
all-or-nothing thinking /
Learn to love food / Know
you are worth it

Grace around food.

—No. 3

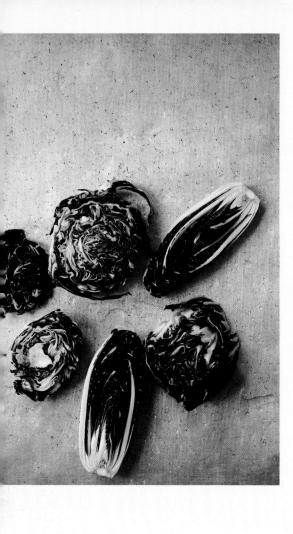

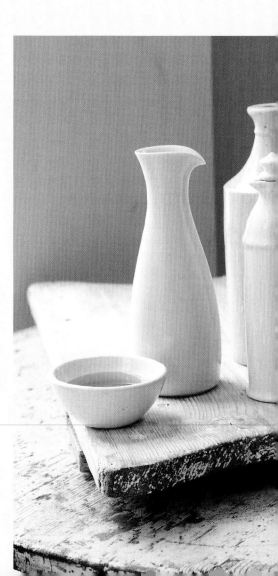

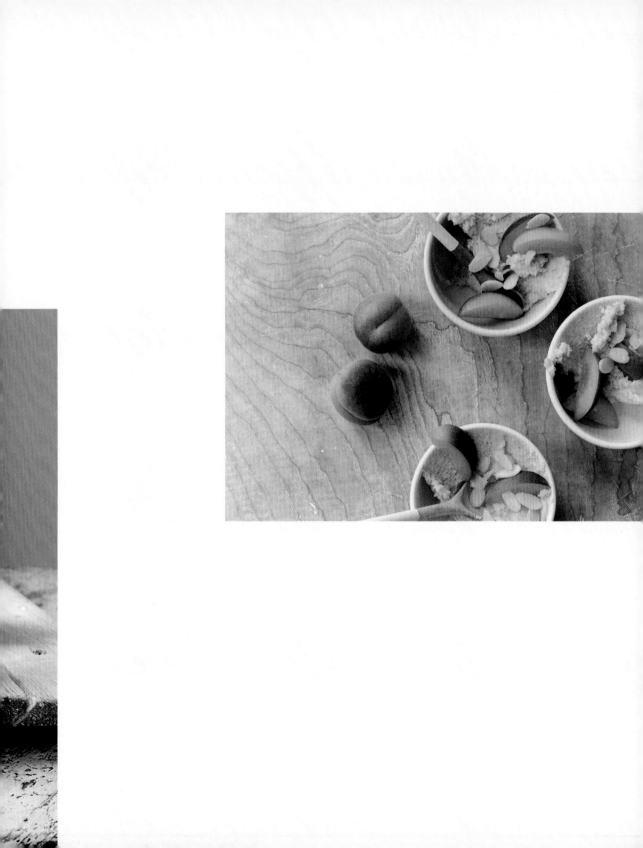

"Indulge in life, not food."

Dana James, Nutritional Therapist, New York

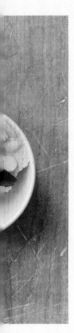

The thinking behind this chapter came about after I began to see a pattern emerging among my clients. Time and time again smart, successful people sat in front of me and admitted variations of the same thing. That after a long day appearing calm and in control of a busy and successful life they collapsed on the sofa and ate chocolate or ice cream until their stomachs hurt, or late at night they would have their heads stuck in the fridge eating anything they could find. These people ran successful businesses and held important positions in large companies. They juggled the demands of raising children and marriage with running a home and a great social life. They knew about nutrition and ate healthily all day. They appeared to glide effortlessly through life looking glamorous and in control. Yet during certain moments of the day they felt utterly helpless around food and ate without grace. They simply stuffed themselves silly. So what was going on?

First of all I want to make it clear that these clients didn't have an eating disorder. If I have clients who do suffer with eating disorders, I always refer them to the appropriate professional because I'm not equipped to give them the help they need. But I do see clients I would describe as emotional eaters, disordered eaters, mindless eaters and so on. Food is so much more powerful than we perhaps acknowledge, not only for its health-giving (or disease-giving) properties, but also for just how much control it can have in our lives. I would say that most people have at some point in their lives used food in an emotional way. This conjures up Bridget Jones–style images of lonely people eating ice cream on their sofa after a break-up. But emotional eating has way many more complexities and facets to it. Some of us "stress eat" at our desks, some "mindlessly eat" while multitasking or vegging out, others are stuck in a binge/diet cycle, or simply eat too much when we are bored or sad. We can overeat as a form of release. A classic way to let off steam is by consuming something whether it's in the pub after work or in the middle of the day when overwhelmed or anxious. When you look at the many scenarios food plays in our lives, it's pretty powerful stuff.

Our relationships with food Let's give food the attention and acknowledgment it deserves. It keeps us alive, literally. Every single cell in our body requires nutrients to function and we get those nutrients from food. We eat to survive, to make energy and to function. If we don't eat food or drink water, we become ill. At this stage let's think about what is, and what isn't food. I have said already that food in its most natural form is all we should eat. When did we lose connection with what is and isn't real food? I often have to explain several times to clients the difference between "food" as in what is sold in package, and real food, as in what grows from the ground, on trees or bushes, swims in the sea or animals we eat for meat. Yet so many of us eat for other reasons—to fill voids, or to distract or alter the way we are feeling. We know that some foods impact the brain in an opiate-like way, so some of us seek that pleasure (from food) to avoid pain (from something going on in our lives).

I recognized quite early on in my career that while I can deliver to clients as much information or inspiration as possible, if they are trapped in an ungraceful, emotional cycle with food that they can't recognize, name or address, they aren't going to be able to make consistent or long-term changes. Not everyone can. I don't have a magic wand to lift away their pain, much as I wish. For some it's a journey, their journey, and it can take a long time to peel away the layers and get their relationship with food under control. While I want it for every client I can't want it more for them than they want it for themselves. It has to be their journey, but the appointments can sometimes be the start even if they don't reach their final destination immediately. The messages we were taught as children around food can play a huge part in how we use food. Being told to be quiet at the table, to finish our plates, be forced to eat foods that we didn't like and coerced with sweet treats at the end doesn't exactly set us up for a celebratory, balanced and happy relationship with food does it? Or being given sweet treats or junk food as a form of love or as a reward or a comfort—a bit of a confusing message that we can still hold on to when we grow up. All of these habits go against everything I say in this book. Yet I meet so many clients whose relationship with food is still wrapped up in their childhoods.

"You are what you eat. So don't be fast, cheap, easy or fake."

What type of eater are you?

You may already be a graceful eater. This means you eat mindfully—you eat when you are hungry and you choose healthy, natural and nourishing foods that you cook with care and eat serenely, eating small mouthfuls and chewing each bite thoroughly. You concentrate on your eating and stop when you are full. You don't eat past the point of satiety, so you never feel uncomfortably full and bloated after eating, or ashamed and guilty. You eat purely to nourish your body and you enjoy your food. If this describes the way you eat, then that's fantastic news. However, if you have yet to find your grace around food, it might help if you first recognize the type of eater you are.

The on/off eater It's so common to go "on" a diet. We start with great intentions and excitement for how we will feel. It can last a few days or a few weeks but then suddenly it gets too hard, too restrictive or something happens to throw us off course. Then, when we are "off" course, we go for it, eating and drinking everything we have missed during the "on" period. Naturally this leads to feeling terrible, usually bloated and tired. Then we decide to have another try "on" this diet or try another diet, always seeking the solution to this yoyo way of eating. There are always new diets appearing with all kinds of tricks and promises to seduce you. It's a "bipolar" way of eating. Boomeranging from green juices to wine and french fries, rarely finding a happy balance, and at what cost to our metabolism? To our confidence? To our blood sugar levels? To our brain health? To our body? I see this pattern so often and it's a miserable place to be—always feeling either like a failure or hungry, and worse, rarely achieving the original goal. Obsessing over calories or fats, denying ourselves or stuffing our faces is not eating with grace, this on/off mentality is a horrid cycle of setting ourselves up for failure; from the yin to the yang—never a balance.

The rushed eater Eating isn't a priority for these types of eaters. Eating is done as quickly and thoughtlessly as possible, usually while doing something else more important like working or traveling. Food is grabbed while replying to emails, in meetings or driving and it's barely registered. Chewing takes too much time despite the bloating and indigestion. I always point out that we don't have teeth in our stomachs—food has to be broken down by the teeth before passing to the stomach. Chewing food properly before swallowing it helps the stomach and digestive juices do the next stage of digestion. If we don't chew properly it's harder work for the gastric juices and this may lead to larger particles of food entering the small intestine, which may reduce nutrient absorption as well as lead to food sensitivities and bacterial overgrowth. The rushed eater usually struggles with IBS symptoms and ultimately will have to slow down one day to undo the damage.

> *The rushed eater usually struggles with IBS symptoms and ultimately will have to slow down one day to undo the damage.*

The stressed eater A sad but consistent state these days, the stressed eater tends to end their day with a four or five hour food onslaught in a way to switch off and escape the non-stop pressures of life. Eating becomes "ME" time and letting off steam is diving into a bag of chips or a package of cookies. There isn't a lack of knowledge about food but there is often an underlying anger about how overwhelming life is and hence a sense of entitlement to eat whatever they want. It might even be healthy food, but just too much of it, and eating in an almost comatose state, trying to slow down from the day but unable to slow the eating until a different state is achieved—usually FULL! Sadly, as much as we may try to fill a void created by stress and overwhelming to-do lists, this is not a successful method to ever undo the effects of stress, and in fact this way of eating only exacerbates it.

The secret eater Eating secretly is equally common. Many of us are virtuous in public while shamefully piling in junk food behind closed doors. From waiting until the house is asleep and raiding the fridge to hitting the gas station and eating it in the car or quickly picking up the children's leftovers. Without realizing, this type of eater consumes way more food than they think and there is usually a lot of guilt and shame around food. In the same way as a child who comes across a cookie jar when their parents aren't looking this kind of eater feels deprived and wants the "treat" but feels so guilty and hence never lets anyone see them doing it.

The comfort eater Very much driven by emotional states, when sad or lonely, angry or scared. Usually foods like ice cream, cake, chocolate or carbs are the go-to substances. Ironically these types of food certainly aren't comforting—they cause blood sugar levels to fluctuate, which causes a crash of energy, creating more hunger and a worse mood. Turning to sugary foods when down has the same effect as drinking alcohol when down—it makes it all so much worse.

The drunk/hungover eater A fine way to sabotage willpower! Alcohol drastically affects blood sugar balance and leads us to be hungrier and then to overeat, especially the day after. I have watched clients undo weeks of healthy habits in one night of boozing. It's so easy to become distracted by a bowl of nuts, crisps or canapés when out socializing, and even without thinking about it to devour the lot. I know I have fallen prey to this!

The distracted eater This is a purely unconscious way of eating, continually grazing. Regardless of what or when it is, if there is food around or offered, it will be eaten, without any thought. If food isn't around, it's not an issue. Dr. Brian Wansink, an American food psychologist from Cornell University in the U.S., has spent much of his career studying the many non-hunger reasons behind our eating decisions. He has found that sometimes it's our environment, and not our emotions, that cause us to overeat. For example, he's discovered that serving food on a large plate or bowl makes us eat more. We consume 22 percent more food on a 12-inch plate than a 10-inch plate. The same goes for glasses. If drinking wine serve it in a smaller glass because Wansink also found that the popular oversized wine glasses that are around now cause us to drink more. He found that eating in front of the TV also causes us to mindlessly eat more.

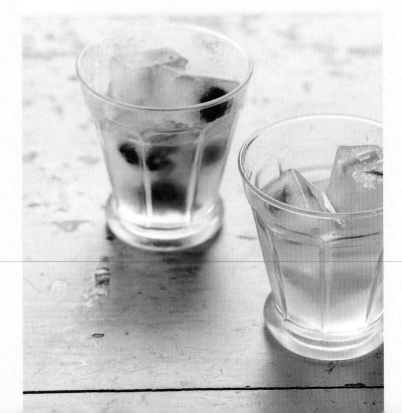

"You're not hungry, you're bored. Drink some water and know the difference."

How to find your grace around food

The previous section shows you some of the many examples that I see, which for simplicity I have put into different categories, but I do see people who overlap with all of them. It's not about being one or the other, it's about how the many different emotions or lifestyles affect how we interact with food. It's not about calories in and calories out nor is it about being lazy or greedy, there are so many different scenarios that fuel how we choose to eat.

So exactly how can you find your grace around food?

Don't give food a label I don't like it when my clients describe food as "good," "bad" or "a treat." For example, a common perception is to see salad as "good" and chips as "bad." So when you are "being good" you eat salad. This reinforces the idea that salad is a good, but rather boring food that you eat when you are being disciplined and virtuous, whereas chips are bad, yes, but delicious and tasty. Labeling something as "bad" makes it more alluring because it's forbidden. As for the word "treat," you are labeling something that makes you uncomfortably full, bloated, overweight and tired as a treat. Why? Think about how chocolate cake really makes you feel. Imagine yourself eating a huge slice of gooey, sweet chocolate cake. Once you have finished it, do you feel light, energized and revived? No, you probably feel a bit sick, maybe bloated and in a sugar coma of tiredness and grogginess. How is that a treat? So stop labeling such foods as treats. Instead of labeling food, see it for what it is—a way of nourishing you, of making you healthier, stronger, happier and more energized. Make every bite work for you—not against you. Choose foods that make you feel good.

Nourish yourself in other ways Find other ways to comfort yourself, to cheer yourself up if you are sad or entertain yourself if you are bored. Do some fun exercise, see a friend, read a book, explore ways to address your stress or sadness. Turning to food to fulfill this job will only perpetuate the cycle so you will be trapped in the sadness or boredom for years to come.

Eat mindfully and consciously This starts from the moment you buy your food. Mindful eating involves choosing nourishing, healthy, seasonal foods. It means experimenting with different recipes and taking pleasure from cooking. It involves sitting down with loved ones—or quietly and without distraction—and really thinking about the food you are putting into your mouth. Smell it, taste it, chew it properly and eat it slowly while savoring every mouthful. The very opposite of this is mindless eating. This involves throwing the same old staples—usually processed convenience food—into your shopping cart. Quickly cooking it in the same old way and eating it in front of the TV, barely pausing for breath. Mindless eating, which is the opposite of mindful and graceful eating involves piling your fork high when you still have food in your mouth, ready to shovel it in. This type of eating can disrupt digestion and cause bloating. It doesn't help you recognize your body's full signals, so you are more likely to overeat. When you mindfully, gracefully eat, and chew food properly and slowly, you feel fuller quicker and know when to stop eating. You will actually start to appreciate and taste food more.

"The strongest factor for success is self-esteem: believing you can do it, believing you deserve it, believing you will get it."

Make eating a priority

You find time to go to the gym before work. You put your all into your job. You make sure you see your friends regularly and you keep your house clean and tidy. But are you putting enough time aside to eat properly? If not, then start making shopping, preparing and eating food a priority. It's the best thing you can do for your health—and if you are healthy you will do a better job elsewhere in your life.

Similarly, make yourself a priority I tell my clients who are mothers to eat how they want their children to eat. They make their children eat lovingly prepared food with greens, yet they grab a quick bowl of pasta for themselves. They don't let their children have too much sugar, yet they eat chocolate and chips most days. They make their children sit down to eat, yet they themselves eat while standing up or sending work emails. Change this—make yourself and your meals a priority that deserve time and thought and share them with your kids, friends or family.

Slow it right down Most of us eat way too fast. It's become part of our busy culture to gulp down food in between a meeting and a drink after work. This is very much tied up with making food a priority and eating mindfully.

Chew your food thoroughly—remember you don't have teeth in your stomach so give your digestion a helping hand by chewing each mouthful until the food becomes a mushy paste.

Don't pile your fork or spoon too high.

Don't eat continuously until all your food has gone.

Put your cutlery down between each mouthful and give yourself time to chew and breathe.

Eat as though you are having dinner with your future parents-in-law for the first time, or as though you are having lunch with your boss for the first time.

Be graceful, eat slowly and don't gobble!

Avoid all-or-nothing thinking Finding your grace around food involves having a healthy balance. Don't deprive yourself because it will probably lead to a spell of bingeing. Instead, keep things simple and graceful. Eat when you are hungry and stop when you are full. Make every bite count by picking healthy, nutritious food that will sustain you, energize you and keep you healthy. Don't waste time worrying about calories—that isn't what graceful eating is about. Instead tune in to your body. When you feed it properly it will feel good. When you don't, it will tell you in multiple ways.

Limit alcohol Alcohol can turn the most graceful eater into a disgraceful one. As I have already discussed, it causes wild blood sugar swings which makes you hungrier than usual, which can then lead to

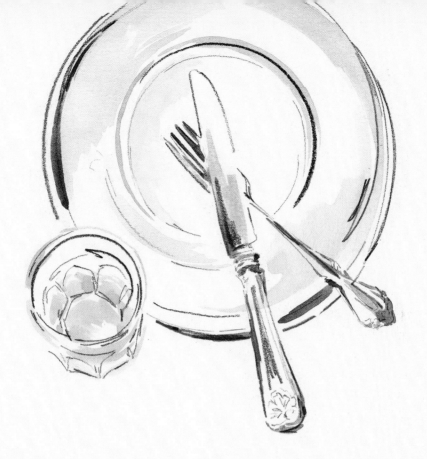

some very ungraceful eating, like buying cheap, processed, greasy junk food and eating it too quickly on your way home from the pub.

Don't use food to change your mood Use food for its true purpose—to guide your health. Don't use it to cheer yourself up, or to cure boredom, stress or loneliness. Turn to other things to help you with that. If you are sad, think about why you are sad and figure out ways to overcome it. Seek the help of a professional to help you unpick the tangled emotions you have around food. If you are stressed, try some breathing techniques or download a mindfulness app. If you are bored, read a magazine, take a bath or do some exercise that you enjoy. Remember that food will never fill a void in your life or mind.

Be prepared I have discussed this in the previous chapter, but I want to remind you how important it is to be prepared when it comes to food. It's very hard to be graceful around food when you get home from work at 8 p.m. to find you have an empty fridge but a package of cookies lying around. When you are hungry and tired, the cookies will win every time and before you know it you will be tucking into them and feeling bad about it. This type of eating isn't graceful, but it isn't surprising either—after all, you are only human. However, if you are prepared and have an organized fridge and freezer full of fresh, healthy and easy to put together food you can trash the cookies.

Don't hold onto weight as a comfort It's very common to stay in our comfort zones. I have had so many clients who appear to want to lose weight but end up sabotaging their efforts, either by losing then regaining or giving up before the real weight falls off. I have heard all of the excuses, such as not having enough time or not being bothered about being slim. There are many real fears in making changes. Often, there are consequences to losing weight.

Will you look stupid if you put it all back again? (Absolutely not—this is your journey, no one else's.)

Will you be able to maintain your new body shape? (Yes, if you lost the weight properly and adopt new eating habits that will become second nature once you get used to them.)

Will your friends or loved ones think you are vain? This last fear is very interesting and very real. I had a client whose family used to tease him whenever he tried to lose weight. He had grown up chubby and his friends and family loved him that way; they were that way too. However well meaning, they would then tease him when he tried to lose weight, probably because they too were fearful of change and perhaps it highlighted that they weren't doing it. As a result he unconsciously self-sabotaged his attempts to lose weight as he didn't like how uncomfortable and conflicting they all became. I have also found that problems come up when one half of a couple

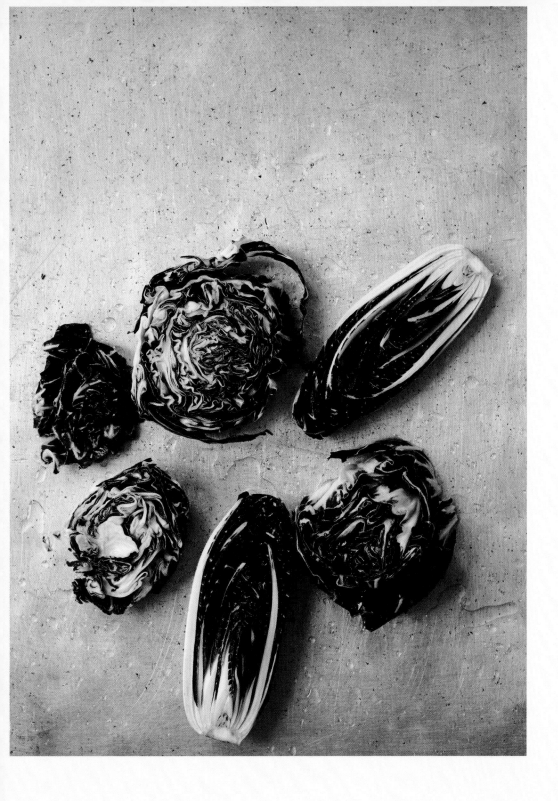

Eat. Nourish. Glow.

loses weight. The non–weight loser may feel threatened about the change, wondering if their new healthy and slim partner will run off with somebody equally healthy and slim, or suddenly they don't have their partner in crime to indulge in overeating with. If you recognize yourself in this description give yourself some credit—you won't fail if you have the right tools in place to eat well. As for what others think, you have to choose your own health and happiness over the thoughts or fears of those around you. Last, don't make weight loss your goal. Instead, aim for more energy, a stomach that doesn't hurt or bloat, clear skin and a happiness and grace around food that doesn't leave you feeling guilty or ashamed.

Learn to love food Every nutritional expert I know loves food. We cherish mealtimes and we enjoy creating recipes and cooking. In fact, after a long day I love to put my phone away, put some music on and just cook for me—it's a form of meditation. There's no reason not to include the kids or your friends or family in this process. I never deprive myself or go hungry, because I know that food is capable of giving me such pleasure. So create happy mealtimes, experiment with cooking and learn to really love food again instead of fearing it—it's life-giving and amazing so don't see it as a chore or something that makes you feel bad, stressed or guilty.

Know you are worth it I often find that some of my clients don't feel worthy of taking the extra time for themselves. They are strong and hardworking, but they don't want to make a fuss about themselves and so settle for far less than they are worth—especially those with families who prioritize their partners or children over themselves. I see mums who lovingly prepare organic meals for their children and insist they sit at the table to eat three times a day, all the while they are sitting there with just a coffee before grabbing a cereal bar as they rush out the door. To those women I urge them to make themselves a priority. Think of it like the oxygen mask warning you get on planes—you have to look after yourself first so you are better able to look after your children. Or as Alcoholics Anonymous say "whatever you prioritize before your sobriety, you stand to lose." I say the same replacing sobriety with health. We can buy beautiful clothes and expensive creams; we can have immaculate homes and well-educated kids, but if we aren't feeding ourselves, or our loved ones properly, then what message is that sending out? We must treat ourselves as we would treat anyone and anything else—with care and love, patience and respect. Nourish yourself because you deserve it.

Be conscious around food, choose nourishment instead of "food." Eat it slowly, savor it, enjoy it, share it and don't eat in a way you would be embarrassed by if others were watching. Ultimately, get in touch with what is the driving force of your relationship with food.

Endless eating / Free yourself from snacking / So, what type of snacker are you? / How to go snack free / Take it one step at a time—it's just one piece of the jigsaw / When snacking is OK / Don't go hungry / Why evening snacking is such a bad idea

Stop snacking.

—*No. 4*

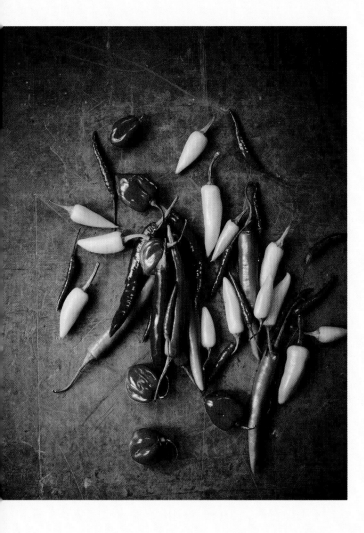
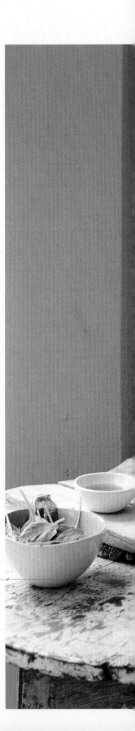

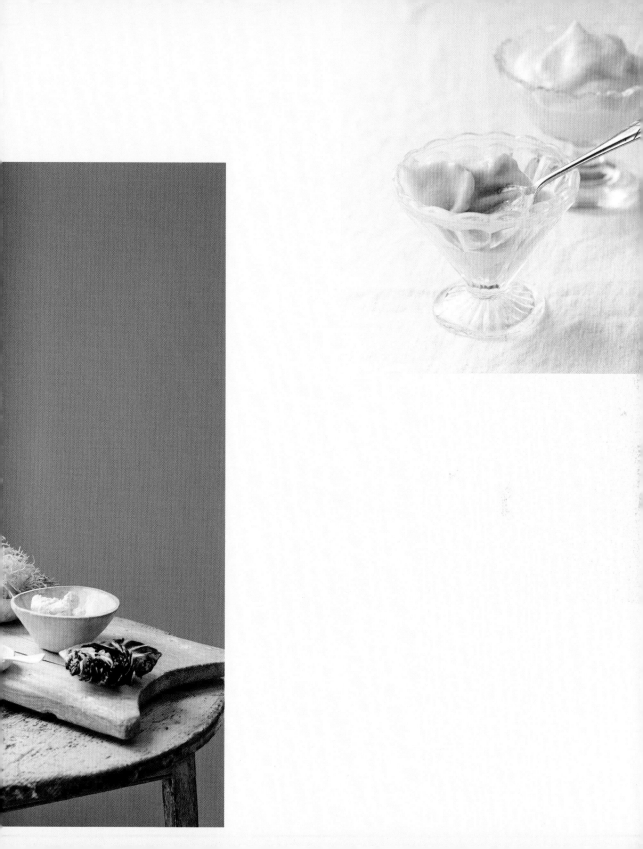

> "The food you eat can be either the safest, most powerful form of medicine or the slowest form of poison."

Ann Wigmore

When I first trained to become a nutritional therapist it was common practice to teach people to eat little and often. Healthy eating was all about managing blood sugar levels—we didn't want them to get too high and so encouraged people to eat the right foods to avoid this, but we also didn't want them to drop too low and hence suggested small healthy snacks. The whole principle of eating a healthy, well-balanced diet was to have three main meals a day plus two or three small snacks in between. I told my clients to eat this way, I ate this way myself and it seemed to work well. It became mainstream advice and to this day most if not all of my clients, when they first come to see me, are having several snacks throughout the day. Some healthy, some not so healthy, but the message currently out there is pretty clear—snacking is good. As ever, food manufacturers have jumped on this message and "handy," "snack-sized" food is available everywhere meaning we can graze throughout the day in the belief it's good for us.

But my views on this changed in 2008 when I went to a lecture about insulin management and pancreatic function. Somewhat controversially he suggested that humans just don't need to snack—especially not as much as they do. Most of the nutritionists in the room—myself included—gasped slightly. This was going against everything we had been taught and was at odds with what we were telling our clients. Surely regular snacking on foods like nuts and fruit kept our metabolism healthy, our blood sugar levels stable and didn't leave us so hungry we were raiding the cookie jar in between meals? It was one of those seminal moments in life when something you believed in for so long is held up and questioned and you suddenly realize that, actually, it might not be true after all. This is the nature of nutritional therapy, as an evolving science we continue to learn more and more. But such is the nature of humans and the media that we jump on a fad or take health knowledge to extremes and hence all of the frustrations people feel about getting mixed messages.

But is no snacking really so new? We know that the human body was not designed to consume a constant supply of food. It was designed to endure regular periods of fasting because hundreds of years ago it had to. Our hunter/gatherer ancestors didn't have a constant supply of sandwiches, cakes and cookies nor even fruit and nuts—sometimes food was plentiful, other times it was sparse. The body is fine with that, but it seems that the modern mind is not. We have convinced ourselves we need to keep grazing and the food manufacturers and supermarkets are only too happy to reinforce this idea (motivated by profits, not by health). As discussed in Chapter Three, we now use food for way more than just fuel, but to suppress emotional states. The truth is: if you are snacking, you are eating more than you need.

Endless eating

Today most of us are exposed to—and encouraged to eat—a constant drip-feed of food, barely going an hour without consuming something. Breakfast followed by a latte on the way to work or after the school run, then an apple mid-morning then more coffee or tea, maybe a cookie or a handful (or a bag!) of nuts. Lunch is followed by a low-fat yogurt, maybe another latte mid-afternoon and more fruit, or perhaps a chocolate bar or a piece of cake if it's someone's birthday. Then pre-dinner is a small snack while making dinner, followed by dinner and then maybe something sweet after dinner and again before bed. Does this sound familiar? It has become a normal day for many, yet it's quite extreme, and far too much food. There are also healthier versions of this scenario that still lead to the consumption of too much food, even good food. Even if you aren't overweight, this amount of food will not be conducive to good health— our digestive system must work to break it down, our liver to sort or eliminate it, our kidneys to filter it, our blood to carry it, our cells to make energy . . . constant eating is constant work for our bodies. It has become easy to eat from the moment we wake until the moment we go to bed, without thinking and using food to prop us up all day long. This is just how I used to eat.

Constant eating will constantly stimulate the production of insulin, an inflammatory hormone that we don't want to have elevated levels of in our bodies. A permanent presence of insulin will put our bodies into fat storage mode. This fat can be visible or invisible but both are damaging to our health. The worst offenders are refined carbohydrates and sugary snacks, but even healthy snacks mean our bodies are constantly working. They aren't designed to function well with an onslaught of too much or too regular food, and if that food is processed and sugary. It's not hard to see why our health is declining.

It is not unusual for me to see people who eat really healthily but can't lose weight or get rid of their bloating, frequent infections or low energy. It's often because they are being let down by their snacking habits. They munch through the day on sugar-filled snack-sized foods, like cereal bars, fruit, green juices and smoothies, chocolate bars, yogurts and bags of nuts. Yes, some of these food choices are healthy but just because something is healthy, like nuts, doesn't mean we can eat the whole bag! I see an almost "snack blindness" where we have no idea we are almost doubling our food intake each day in snacks alone.

But back to the lecture that inspired this chapter. Up until the day I attended the lecture, I had eaten little and often. My snacks were healthy and sensibly sized, but this information was too powerful to ignore. So the next day I thought, "Right, I've got to try this." I would like to add here that I'm in no way a fan of fad diets; I never go hungry; I never starve myself and I never worry about calories or dress sizes. I'm balanced and practical about food and my goal is always health—and not weight loss.

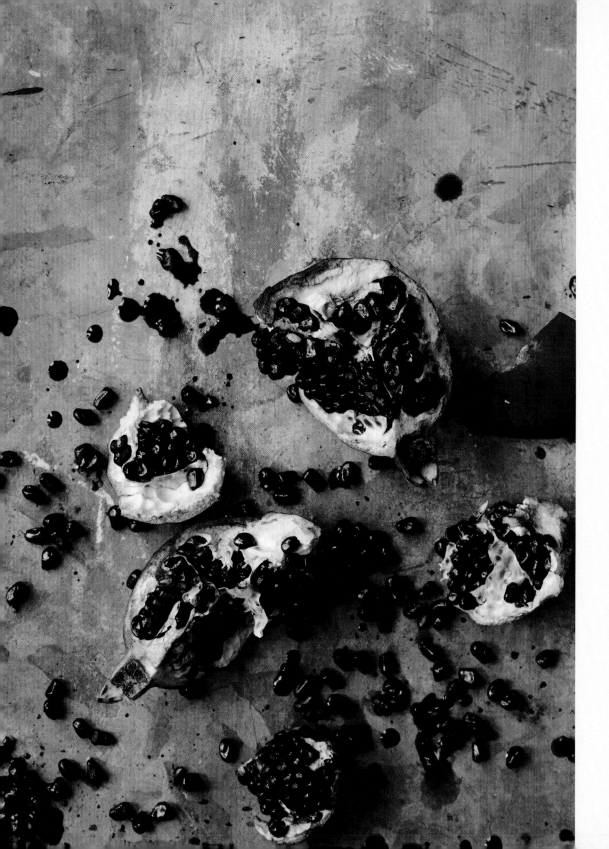

Eat. Nourish. Glow.

Free yourself from snacking

I can't ignore the science, so I gave up snacking. It was hard—my body had been trained to expect food every three hours. I also had teas or green juices so a few hours after breakfast I felt hungry and quite uncomfortable. It was a combination of my mind seeking out distraction but also my body feeling physically hungry. I was still having a fairly low-fat breakfast of oatmeal, fruit and flaxseeds back then, but I realized I needed good healthy fats at breakfast to make the transition to no snacking more easily. I started having avocado and salmon, or poached eggs and greens or even sometimes a chicken and avocado salad for breakfast and within a few days my body adapted and I was able to go happily snack free until lunch. It's a liberating way to eat.

For a start, it gave me freedom from food. Whereas before I was either eating meals, snacking, thinking about food or preparing food, when I gave up snacking I felt liberated. I was eating exactly what I needed to nourish myself at mealtimes, so I never felt hungry or deprived. I felt really good eating this way—less work for my digestive system so less bloating and better energy. Most importantly I had complete confidence in my ability to go without food for a few hours. Remember, humans are designed to fast for periods—there are popular diets based on intermittent fasting, where you eat normally for five days and cut back for two days which are based on this science. But I don't advocate ever eating what you want on some days and not on others as this isn't focusing on the quality of the food eaten. Surely, it's better to strive for consistency each day and cut out the snacks? I went snack free around the same time as I gave up gluten and I believe that these were two of the best changes I ever made for my health.

116

"Every time you eat or drink, you are either feeding disease or fighting it."

Heather Morgan, MS, MLC

So, what type of snacker are you?

Before you decide to give up snacking it's worth knowing what kind of snacker you are as this will help make your transition to no snacking easier. The following are the most common types I see among my clients . . .

The mini-meal snacker I don't advocate calorie counting, but if you are having mini meals for your snacks then you are most likely stacking up the calories. Five or six rice cakes with cheese or a spread or a whole bag of nuts is a mini meal—this constantly elevates insulin.

The "healthy" snacker The mistaken belief that you simply can't overeat a healthy food such a fruit or fruit smoothies—you can.

The "association" snacker This snacker is seduced by the food industry and by marketing campaigns—low-fat yogurt, fat-free chips or "skinny" muffins, cookies with tea, chocolate at the gas station—always a snack for a situation. The amount of people I meet who just can't allow themselves out of their food comfort zones—they have their habits and eating anything other than cereal for breakfast is just too "weird." WHO

SAYS YOU CAN'T EAT BROCCOLI for breakfast? It's merely pre-conditioning. We have been told that Cocoa Krispies is a natural breakfast choice, but by becoming mindful about food habits and eating to nourish your body—not "just because" is the start. This phrase is often used by clients when I ask them why they buy a chocolate bar when in line for gas. Or why they have a cookie with their tea. Ask yourself if you are truly hungry, if you really need that food. Don't be a "just because" eater.

The meal skipper Trying to lose weight or just too busy, meals are skipped as much as possible and a good day is a day when only a few snacks have been consumed instead of meals. Or merely a busy day where main meals have been missed but a muffin was grabbed and eaten on the go then a bar of chocolate and chips later in the day. If you eat structured meals containing fat, protein and plants then you won't find yourself in these situations. Make eating a priority, like you do other things in your life. And plan—if you often work through lunch then you need to start bringing your lunch to work.

The leftover snacker Sound familiar to the mums out there? It's so easy to eat the children's leftovers because you don't like waste or the food looks too good to throw away. Sometimes because you have prioritized your child's food, you have forgotten about your own and only had a coffee. While I hate the waste of food, don't be a human garbage pail. Be mindful and only eat food when you are actually hungry not just because it's there. If you don't trust yourself around leftovers throw them away immediately or save them for the following day.

The bored snacker This type snacks in front of the TV or on a long flight. They don't do it because they are hungry; they do it because they are bored. If you are this type of snacker then read Chapter Five, which deals with boredom eating. Remember, don't eat to suppress an emotion; eat mindfully because you are hungry and need nourishment.

The social snacker While I love eating with friends and family and urge all my clients to sit down and enjoy mealtimes with their loved ones, I'm aware that social situations sometimes make us overeat when we don't need to. Canapés, parties and buffets can be treacherous turf for snackers. We graze continuously on food simply because it's there and because it's the social thing to do. I'm not saying to never enjoy the lovely canapés or the buffet—do, but savor the taste, the smell, the occasion and be mindful about just how much you actually need to eat.

The office snacker Office life is a snacking minefield. The many constraints of office life from looking for distraction to working through lunch or simply the office camaraderie when the cake goes around makes it a battle zone for anyone wanting to change their eating habits and focus on their health. It starts with awareness, then eating right so that when faced with temptation you are able to think about if you really want or need it.

How to go snack free

I don't advise clients to go cold turkey with snacks. It's essential to get a few things in place first to make the smooth transition. Sometimes I will start by giving clients healthy snacks and once their blood sugar has stabilized, then I begin to remove the snacks and really clean up their diet. Here's how to do it . . .

It must start with eating the right meals. Skipping meals or eating processed, high-sugar junk food is like taking away the scaffolding too soon. With the best will in the world, it's not laying down the right foundations to make this change. You won't be able to do it if you eat too little at mealtimes—if you just have sugar or carbs at breakfast, you won't be able to last without snacking until lunchtime—this means a green juice as much as it means Special K. You need fat and protein with your breakfast as well as vegetables and a portion of fruit. I'm not meaning to overeat until you are stuffed, but a proper breakfast. Every meal should be made up of these three things—fat, protein and plants. A meal purely consisting of refined carbohydrates, like a bowl of pasta, will cause havoc with your blood sugar levels and leave you hungry (most likely for sugar) an hour later and make giving up snacking nearly impossible. Don't go fat free either—if you are having salad for lunch or dinner you need some good fat such as avocado or seeds with it (along with protein of course).

If you eat the right thing at mealtimes your blood sugar levels will remain steady several hours after eating.

Start slowly. It's very hard to stop all snacks straight away unless your diet is very good. If a new client comes to see me and they are eating cereal for breakfast and a sandwich for lunch, followed by a pasta or rice dish for dinner, I work on their meals first and worry about cutting out snacks later. Clients—and readers—like this are far better off eating little and often until they improve their meals. Only then should they attempt to give up snacking.

Before you snack, ask yourself why you are doing it. This goes back to the core of this book—mindfulness. Be mindful and ask yourself if you are really hungry and need that snack or if you are simply eating to suppress and avoid another emotion.

Be mindful and ask yourself if you are really hungry and need that snack or if you are simply eating to suppress and avoid another emotion.

Don't be scared of feeling hungry. I'm not advocating feeling faint and starving, of course not, this is equally detrimental to our health, but being a little hungry and ready for your meals is not a bad thing. It's merely our minds that are uncomfortable with this state. I never go hungry, but I'm not scared of feeling the first gentle pang of hunger either. It's very normal now to be unaware of what genuine hunger even feels like because we have got so used to the state of being completely full, most of the time. Children often have an instinctive, primal way of eating that's in tune with how our ancestors used to eat. They don't need the clock to tell them when to eat—their body tells them.

Take it one step at a time. Giving up snacking—much like every other part of this book—is one small piece of a jigsaw. If you don't get the hang of it right away, don't worry. Everything will come together naturally when it feels right. If somebody had told me years ago that I wouldn't eat sugar, nor snack, nor drink endless cups of tea every day I'd think to myself, "How on earth am I going to manage all that?" But I do and it seems so effortless because I have taken each step slowly. I didn't make all these changes overnight. I found what worked for me as I've gone along and while no snacking works for me, it might not work for you, as I'll explain next.

When snacking is OK

Although I don't advocate snacking, there are some occasions that call for it. If you are stuck at work at 7 p.m. and haven't had dinner, then I would recommend you snack. If you are traveling and changing time zones, then snack. Naturally, I would encourage that the snacks are real foods such as fruits, nuts and seeds—not the "Packages and Promises" in Chapter Two. If I do snack, apple slices with hazelnut or almond butter, or cherry tomatoes with walnuts, or avocado slices mashed with seeds and lemon are just a few of the things I enjoy.

If you are genuinely hungry between meals—and I mean hungry, not bored or looking for a distraction—then have a snack. Don't go hungry, but keep it small and look at your meals and see if they can be improved upon or increased slightly, so you don't need to snack after the next one.

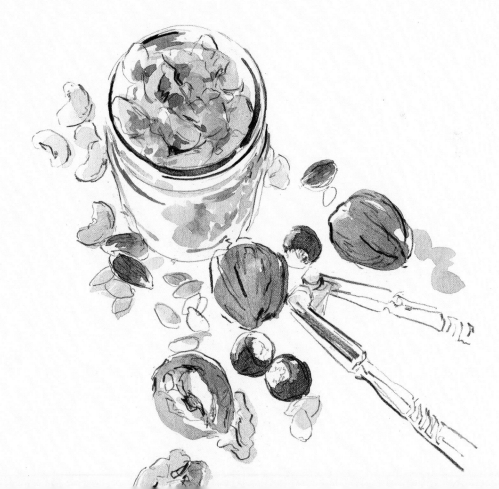

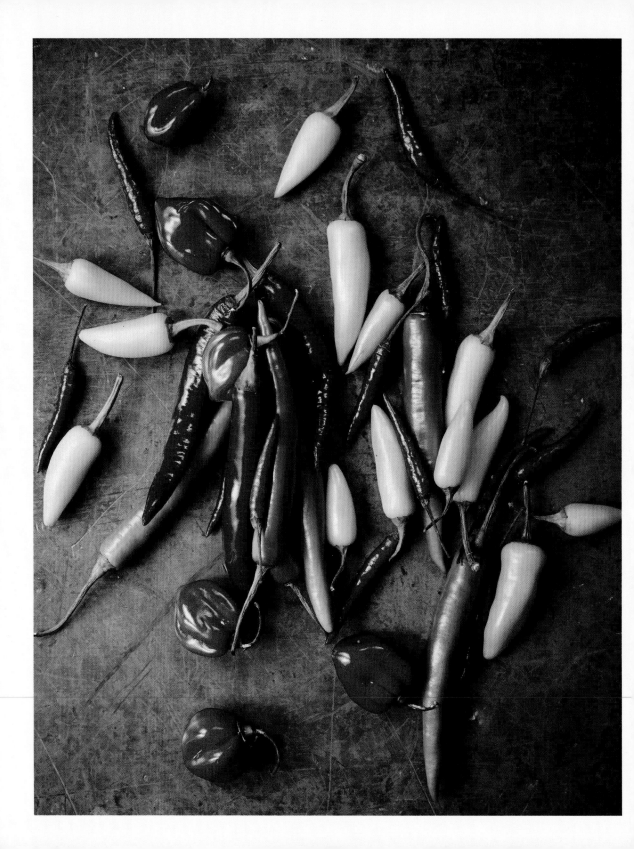

Last, why evening snacking is such a bad idea

As I said at the start of this chapter, we know that the human body doesn't need a constant supply of food. It needs a break and this is especially true overnight. One of the most important things you can do for your health and metabolism is to fast for 12 hours overnight. Now, this seems simple enough. After all, we are asleep for most of this time, but so many of us snack between finishing dinner and the moment we go to bed. Our metabolisms are hard wired to expect a nightly fast—TV and evening snacking weren't an option for our hunter/gatherer ancestors. Food eaten between 8 p.m. and midnight is most likely to be sugary and processed because mindless snacking reaches a peak in the evening when we are exhausted from the day and slumped in front of the television. It's also when we are sleepy and our willpower is running low. So stop eating after dinner and don't eat again until breakfast.

CHAPTER 4 · IN A NUTSHELL

Start by improving your meals, then improve your snacks. Finally, make your meals so healthy, nourishing and balanced that you don't need snacks at all.

Why perfect doesn't work / A word of warning / Watch habit-forming practices / Flip your thinking—remember everything you do is a choice / How to create habits, not restrictions / Making new habits—why "treats" will slowly start to lose their appeal

Be consistent, not perfect.

—No. 5

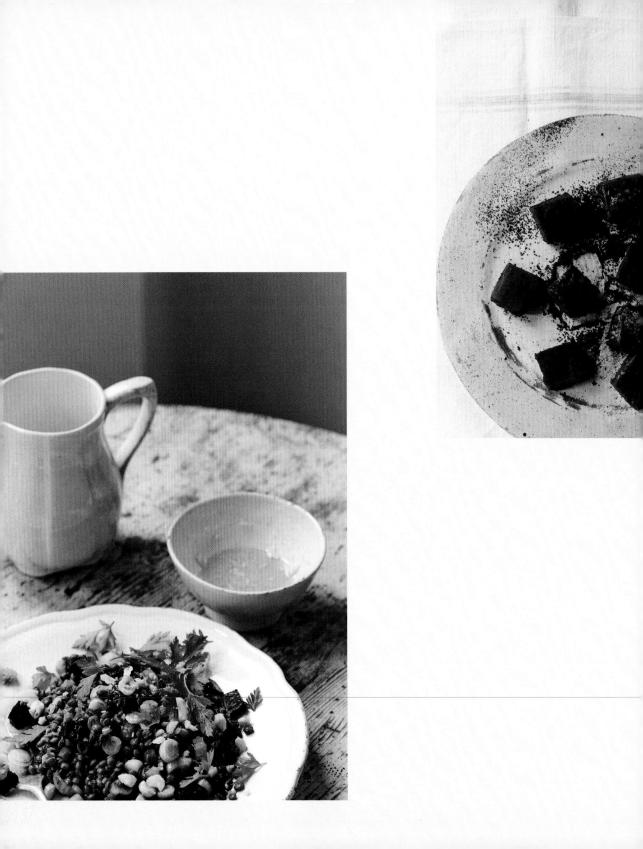

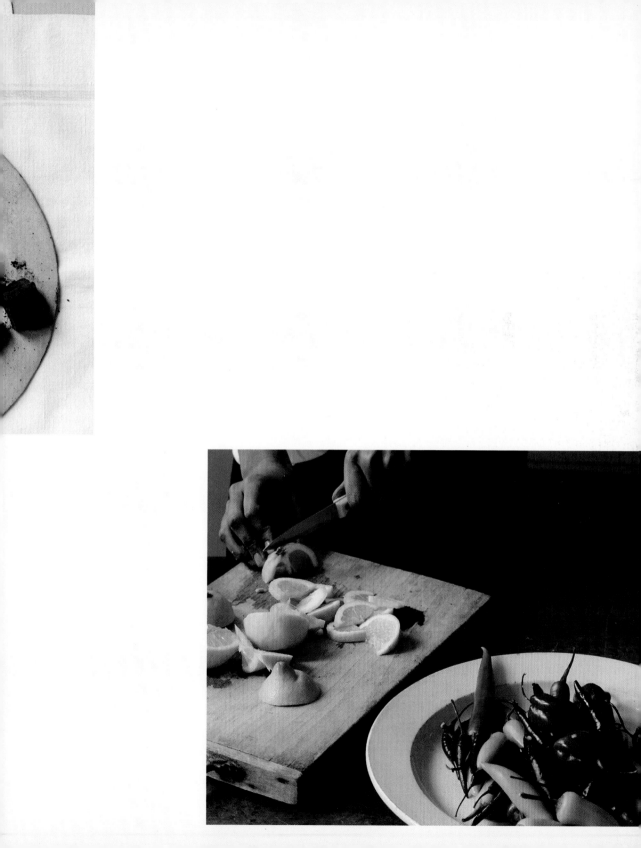

"Create healthy habits, not restrictions."

I love the title of this chapter. It's something I regularly tell my clients and it's a concept I try to apply to my life. Because being consistently "good" but knowing it's OK not to be perfect is one of the most liberating things you can do for your body and mind.

I didn't always realize this. When I first started out as a nutritional therapist I was very hard on myself. I couldn't make all the changes to my diet that I wanted to at once and I felt ashamed and berated by my lack of willpower. I expected perfection from the outset and the pressure I put on myself was immense. But slowly, I realized that good habits take time to form. As I worked with more and more clients, I saw just how hard everyone finds it. So instead of making lots of changes overnight, I made them gradually and went easy on myself in the process. If I slipped up that was OK. This way of thinking boosted my confidence and helped me to make more changes. Striving for perfection, on the other hand, dented my confidence, which made me want to give up altogether.

It's the same with my clients. If they berate themselves for having a piece of cake or a beer, pretty soon they will lose confidence in their ability to make changes to their life, assuming they are not up to it, and then they will give up altogether. The same happens if I berate them when they tell me they have gone off track. I don't make any fancy promises that I can transform their health, but I give them the necessary information and tools so they can make more informed choices—it's up to them. I also give them the freedom not to be perfect. I have found over the years that giving my clients the green light to eat what they want when they feel the need to actually takes the appeal out of that food. One of my clients recently texted me to confess he was in a restaurant and he had just ordered a pizza. "Good for you," I replied, "I hope it tastes delicious." He'd been making fantastic progress, losing weight, getting healthy and I didn't want to make him feel guilty as he had already made the decision. A pizza here or there isn't a huge issue (providing you aren't gluten sensitive) but it's the aftermath or the continuation that's the problem. The next time I saw him he admitted that it didn't even taste that great and how he felt the next day just wasn't worth it. His taste buds were used to healthy, fresh, delicious ingredients and as a result the pizza tasted greasy and bland. He had also experienced what it felt like not to be bloated and foggy all the time.

One of two things happens when you are consistently good. Like my client, you may find that when you eat well most of the time you suddenly feel very bloated and uncomfortable when you eat something more processed, greasy or sugary than you have been used to. You quickly remember you don't like feeling this way and go back to eating normally. You quickly realize you don't like fatty, sugary or processed tastes any more. Alternatively, you might enjoy it and find that the occasional slipup doesn't affect you at all. Sometimes a client will be doing really well and then have a night out with friends where they eat a huge bowl of pasta and drink too much wine. They feel fine the next day and the scales don't shoot up. When you are eating well the majority of the time your body can cope with a slipup. What it can't cope with is daily bad habits that accumulate over time to leave you overweight, bloated, tired or sluggish.

Why perfect doesn't work

One of the reasons so many diets fail is that people can only do something restrictive for so long. This is especially true of extreme, restrictive diets that leave you hungry or expect a lot of effort, expensive ingredients or fussy recipes. And of course, we live in the real world where we will be exposed to birthday dinners with friends, family gatherings, slices of cake and glasses of wine. Vowing never to eat these things for life is setting yourself up for failure—and a lifetime of feeling like you are missing out. I think healthy habits should be formed gradually, but kept for life. Make one change at a time, see how it works for you, and then make another.

Don't think of yourself as being on "a diet" because you are not. You can eat whatever you want—I'm not here to tell you what to do, I'm just here to tell you what's worked for me and for many of my clients, and it could work for you too. I'm also a realist and it's OK to let your hair down occasionally. I most certainly do.

This can be a revelation to many of my clients. They come to me at first with an all or nothing attitude to dieting. When they talk to me about their history with food I find they have been having spells of being incredibly disciplined followed by binges and splurges. They mistakenly think that once they have eaten a cookie they may as well have another, then another, then another. There is no point in eating it with negativity and self-loathing flooding through your veins. If you do have it, then enjoy it. Perhaps it's about negotiation with yourself so that you can enjoy a treat but not punish yourself afterward and that in time you and your body will come to learn how to moderate your treats and with that comes an enormous sense of pleasure.

I'm quite strict with clients who come to me with a need to be perfect, because it traps them in such a negative cycle. I went on holiday recently and indulged in red wine and lots of french fries! There are some things that I just wouldn't ever eat like processed meals or sandwiches but I don't have a harsh or fearful interaction with food either, and french fries and wine work for me! Gluten and trans fats don't. We all have our things—there is no one diet for all of us, so it's a case of working out what will and won't work for you and your health goals—be consistent but not perfect.

"It's never too late in the day to start eating better. Have a bad morning? Make an amazing afternoon."

A word of warning

Despite everything I have discussed, you do need to avoid using the "I'm only human" concept as an excuse to hold onto bad habits. It's all too easy to make great headway and lose excess weight, form new habits, get more energy and relief from nagging symptoms and then relax, and slowly but surely veer off track . . . day by day, more and more of the old, negative habits start to creep back in and before long the sugary foods and snacks are suddenly part of your life again and the perfection is the occasional bit of broccoli. I encourage you to get to know where you can slip up and identify what sends your blood sugar rocketing and your willpower wild. There is such a difference between enjoying something occasionally and it becoming a habit. I used to drink so much sugary tea that I don't think I actually registered it—it was just my habit. Now I have one or two cups a week, without sugar and I relish them.

Flip your thinking

It's key to know that everything we do is a choice. There are, however, "food-like substances" available to buy which dramatically affect the food choices we make i.e. they are addictive and cause addictive behavior around them. We all have a choice if we buy these things in the first place, and we can decide how much we want to make food a stressor in our life, emotionally or physically. Choosing a slice of pizza or a piece of cake is your choice and for you to decide if it makes you feel well or unwell. When I first started out I told myself I couldn't have that bag of chips. But as

It's key to know that everything we do is a choice.

we all know, making something forbidden makes it more tempting and I wanted it more. So I tried to talk myself out of it. I had constant, exhausting head chatter going on with myself. I realized that banning something just creates an emotional tug with it—it becomes all you can think about. So I started being more mindful. I began looking at a bag of chips and thinking, "Do I really want them? Do they really taste as good as I'm building up in my head?" I then tried one and really thought about it, and honestly, no they just don't taste as good as I used to think they did. I occasionally eat them now but they always leave me feeling quite uncomfortable—they are just no longer the treat that fresh strawberries are to me now. A recent study from Stanford University in the U.S. found that our brains start to associate certain foods with reward and pleasure. It has little to do with their taste. We want them because our brain is tricking us into thinking that they are tastier than they are. The solution is to be mindful about them, so we out-think this process. Trust me, a bowl of ice cream never tastes as good as the sight, smell and thought of it.

I also ask myself how a certain food makes me feel. Take a bag of chips, for example—instead of looking at the chips and thinking how delicious and crunchy they look, I see them as a bag of greasy, fried food sprinkled with a lot of salty, fake, toxic flavor that will make my stomach bloat and become gassy. One of my clients was hooked on fizzy drinks and would drink several cans of cola a day. I explained to her how chemical and unnatural they are and that she may as well be drinking something from the cupboard under her sink. After this conversation she said she looked at those drinks in a completely different way. I didn't tell her not to drink them; I just questioned why she would want to. It worked. She no longer sees fizzy drinks as delicious or hydrating—she merely sees them as fake, toxic, processed sugar water that is one of the contributing factors to her poor health. She's flipped her way of thinking and doesn't crave them any more.

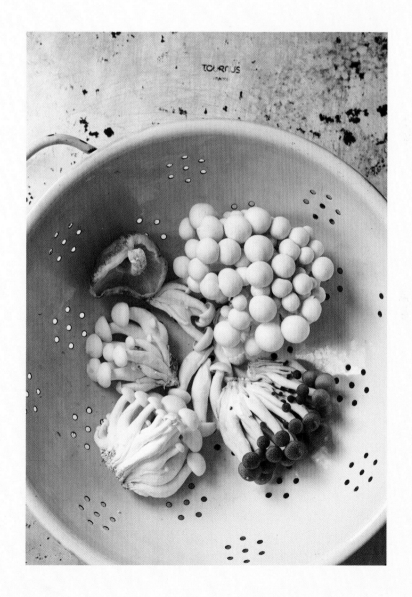

"We become what we want to be by consistently being what we want to become each day."

Richard G. Scott

How to create habits, not restrictions

Much of our eating and drinking is born out of habit. It's not that we prefer a sugary cup of tea and a bowl of cereal for breakfast to a homemade green juice and poached eggs. It's just that we are in the habit of having the tea and cereal. We mindlessly buy the same foods every week in the supermarket without even thinking about it so when it comes to mealtimes we have the same thing in our cupboards, regardless of how it makes us feel. Hopefully this will change after reading Chapter Two and detoxing your kitchen. The point I'm trying to make is that most of our food choices are merely habits and routine—and knowing this is a powerful tool that will help you begin to create healthier new habits. Creating new habits is largely down to being more mindful.

It's also about stepping out of your comfort zone and turning your old habits on their head. Here's an example. One of my clients used to eat two or three slices of toast with low-fat spread for breakfast every day. Every morning he did the same thing without even thinking about it. He felt tired a lot of the time and was snacking right up until lunch—something I put down to his high carb/low-fat breakfast. He left the house early for work so he didn't have time to make a juice or cook some eggs. I sensed that it might have been the wheat as well as the lack of protein that was contributing to his tiredness, so I suggested that he replace the toast with rice cakes and add a sliced tomato, some avocado, pesto and arugula for breakfast instead. He looked at me as if I was crazy. How on earth can you have arugula and pesto for breakfast? It had been so ingrained in him— indeed, it's been ingrained in most of us—that breakfast either consists of cereal, toast or eggs. Things like salad are for lunch, surely? But it doesn't have to be that way. You can eat anything you like for breakfast. When I saw him the following week he told me that it was the most delicious breakfast he had ever had and even his young children loved it. It took no time to prepare, it was tasty and it left him feeling great all morning. He said he could never imagine going back to his old bland slices of toast. He had opened his mind, created a new habit and that was it—he had made a great step in the right direction and it didn't even feel like much of an effort.

Making new habits My clients find that when they start to create new healthy habits—rather than mindlessly reaching for foods "just because"— they never look back. They wake up feeling energized, they feel clean and light during the day, and their sugar cravings subside. They get such an endorphin hit from their new healthy habits and wonder why they persisted so long in their old ways, feeling tired and overweight all the time, and thinking that was normal. When they eat chocolate or drink a fizzy cola drink they are horrified by how sugary it tastes. Their taste buds—which have previously been dominated by all the sugar and fake flavors pumped into processed foods—change and they realize how great nourishing, healthy food tastes. This could happen to you in a matter of days as well.

New habits usually take between a week and a month to kick in. If you are prepared (see Chapter Two) and open minded, then it will happen quickly. Sometimes you may find that some of your old foods you miss are too much to give up—that certainly happens a lot. There's usually one thing that my clients just can't give up, like wine, lattes or bread. With me, it's red wine—I can happily go without chips, chocolate, cakes and bread, but I enjoy red wine when I'm socializing with friends. And I can because it doesn't give me any symptoms (unless I drink too much of course!). One of my clients was the same about her lattes. She was happy to forgo

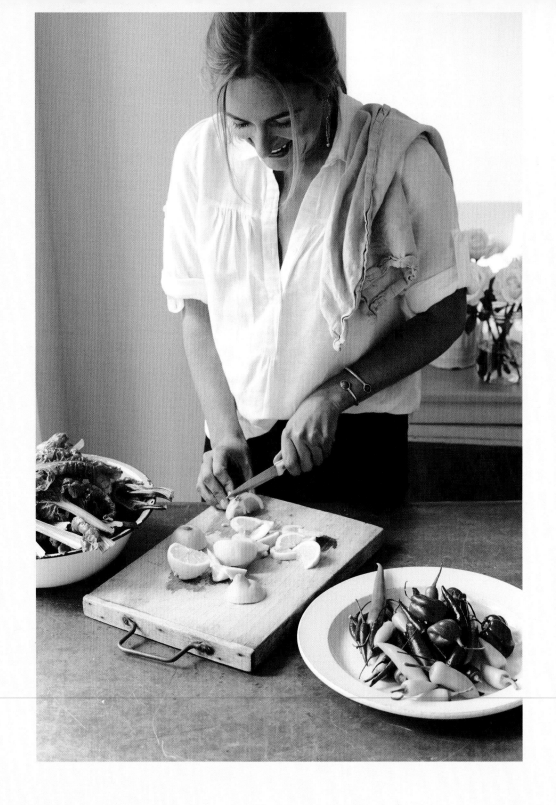

Eat. Nourish. Glow.

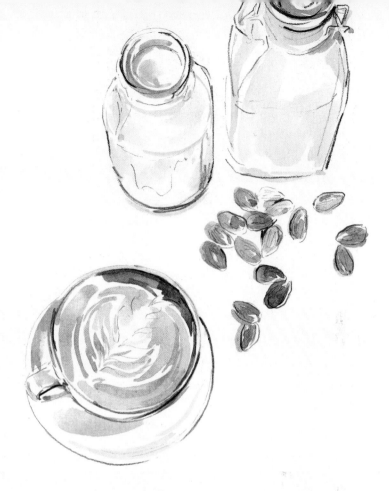

alcohol, sugar, chips, pasta and bread but the one thing she wanted every morning was her latte on the way to work. So we factored this in—she has almond milk latte without the sugar and she absolutely loves it. If a client loves pasta and their body copes OK with the gluten, then they still have it. I do suggest that all new clients go gluten-free for a short while because they are usually suffering with some kind of symptoms and I feel it's beneficial for everyone to experience a break from gluten, to see how they feel. There are multiple alternatives to cooking without gluten and I don't mean all of the processed gluten-free products. I mean things like:

Zucchini Bolognese

Make some zucchini spaghetti with a spiralizer (see page 78). Blanch it in hot water, rinse under cold running water and give it a good shake to dry it. Make your favorite Bolognese sauce using organic low-fat ground beef, tomatoes, onions and mushrooms and stir it through the zucchetti in a pan until hot. Drizzle with a little olive oil and serve immediately.

Celeriac cottage pie

Make a cottage pie in the regular way—shallow-fry some good-quality, grass-fed organic ground meat. Add carrots, onions, peas, mushrooms and homemade vegetable stock. Boil and mash some celeriac with a little olive oil and use as your topping. Bake for around 10 minutes until slightly golden on top.

Why "treats" will slowly start to lose their appeal

I can vouch for the changes that occur to our taste buds and habits when we change the foods we eat. It's not immediate but it happens. What we think we love can very quickly be turned around. When you break the bad habits you realize that actually those "treat" foods don't taste so good after all—and it's a lovely feeling.

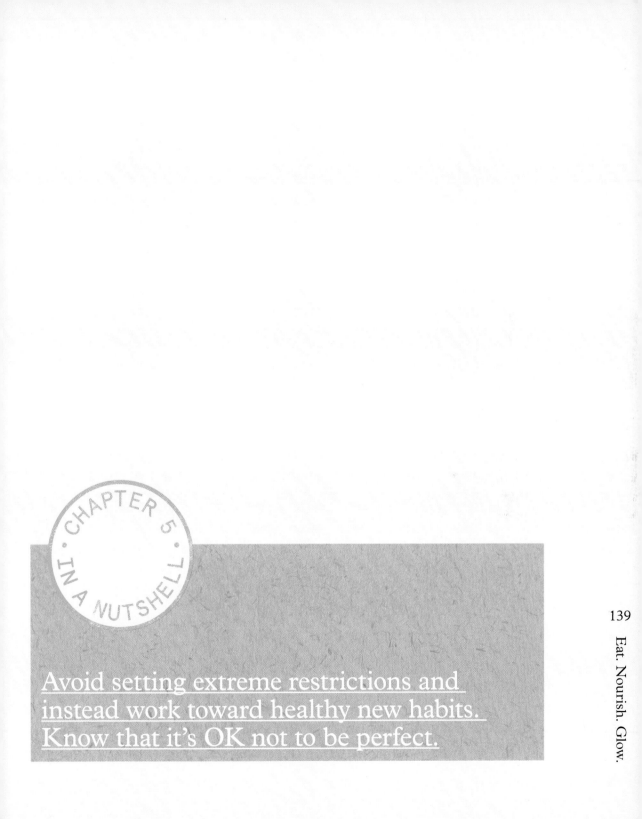

Avoid setting extreme restrictions and instead work toward healthy new habits. Know that it's OK not to be perfect.

Why fat is actually OK /
All fats are not bad for you /
Good fats for your diet /
The real diet villain—sugar /
The sugar rollercoaster ride /
Break the sugar cravings /
Where you will find sugar

Make fat your friend (and sugar your enemy).

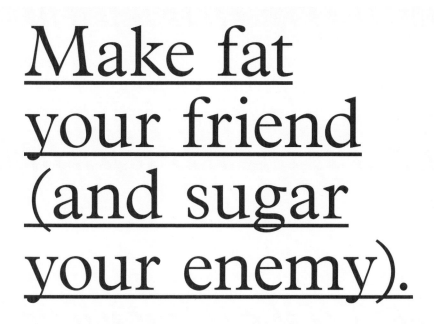

—No. 6

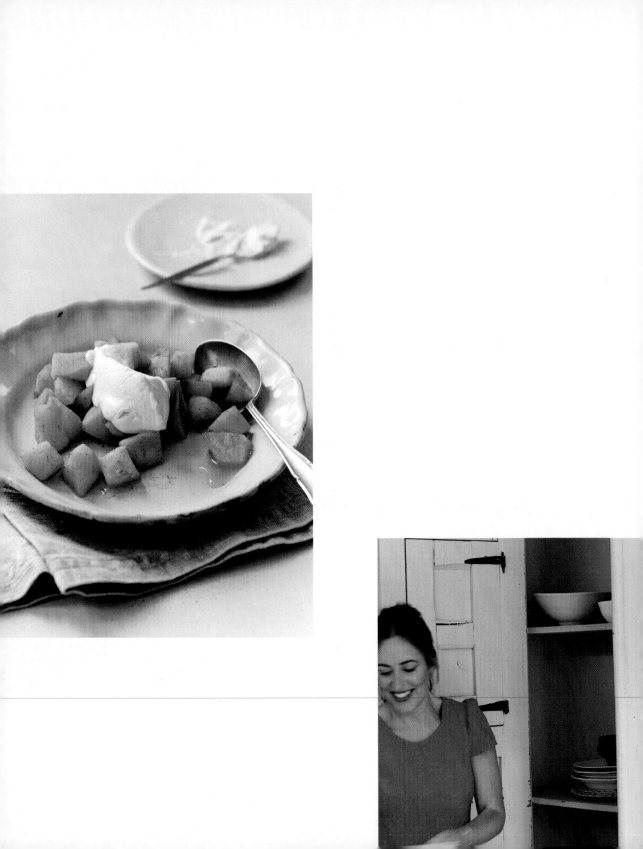

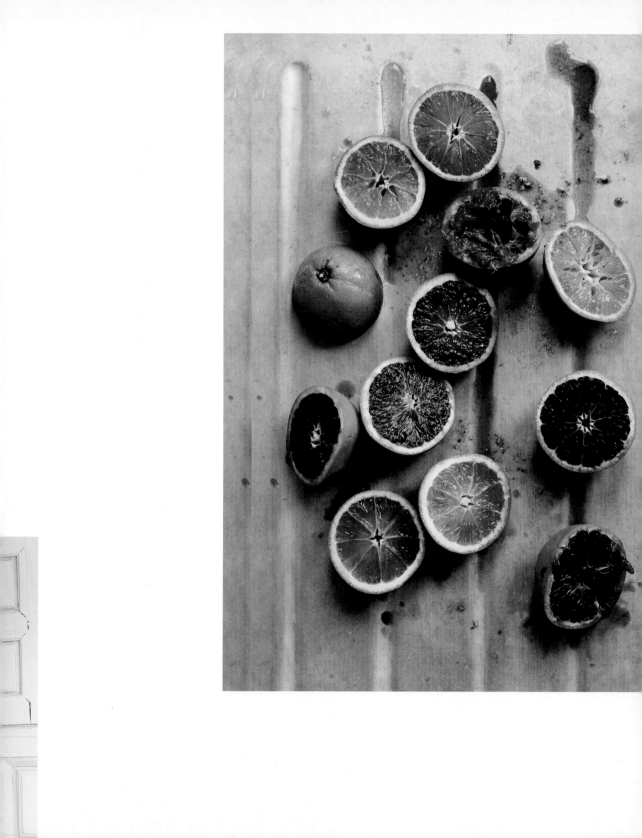

"There are too many people counting calories and not enough counting chemicals."

Fat. It's such an emotive word isn't it? For most of us it conjures up images of greasy food or bulging weight. It's used as an insult and something we have feared to eat.

Rewind 50 years and the average person didn't really know or care about the fat in their food. It was the post-war era and people were just happy to have enough food on the table. They enjoyed home-cooked food bought from their local butcher, baker and grocer and they didn't give a thought to how much fat or calories their food contained.

Then the Eighties delivered a new obsession with fat—or rather, a lack of it. Pure butter was ditched in favor of a bright yellow spread called margarine under the promise that it was a healthier substitute. Full-fat milk from the milkman—where the cream rose to the top of the glass bottle—was replaced with skim milk in plastic containers from the supermarket. Homemade meals of fresh meat and veggies were swapped for low-fat microwave meals from plastic trays or pasta and a ready-made sauce.

Home-baked seasonal fruit desserts were abandoned and bright pink flavored diet mousses took their place, and warm loaves of bread from the baker down the road (that turned stale after a day) were scrapped for sliced bread in plastic wrapping that lasted a week. Calorie counting, "fat-free," "low-fat" and "lite" became diet buzzwords in households all over the country. We were led to believe that we were being fantastically healthy when in reality we were being anything but . . .

This is all due to flawed science and thinking. First, in the 1950s, we were encouraged by the Government to start consuming vegetable oils, which were added to packaged foods, such as margarine and mayonnaise. In the 1960s, health officials advised us that consuming fat increased our risk of heart disease and made us fat, so we began to fear natural foods like butter, red meat and eggs.

Despite the flawed science, the food industry seized upon this wonderful profit-making opportunity and began churning out low-fat versions of everything. Under the guise of making our lives easier and our bodies healthier, low-fat processed foods like yogurts, mousses, sauces in jars, boil-in-the-bag meals, microwavable meals and fruit juices became the new kitchen staples of households everywhere. More chemicals, hydrogenated (damaged) fats and sugar snuck into our homes, and eggs at breakfast were replaced with sugary cereals. Roast beef was out and pasta with a low-fat sauce was in. In 1980, Philip Handler, the president of the National Academy of Sciences in the U.S., described these changes as a "vast nutritional experiment." Did it work? Well in 2014—the year I'm writing this book—we are fatter and sicker than ever, so I think it's safe to answer that question with a resounding "No."

The message about fat being bad was misleading. We didn't increase our fruit and vegetable intake as we were advised, but upped our carbohydrate intake (which was also advised) instead, and a lot of these carbs were the new processed and sweetened kind. We were eating less fat than ever before, but we were getting fatter and with detrimental impacts on our health.

While there's nothing wrong with naturally low-fat foods (fish, chicken, vegetables, etc.), there's plenty wrong with processed low-fat foods. The types of food that started being mass-produced had the fat taken out and sugar, sweeteners and additives put in. Low-fat yogurts, margarines, spreads, low-fat ready-made meals, breakfast cereals, cereal bars and juices are all technically low in calories, but that doesn't mean they won't make you overweight. We know that excess sugar gets converted to fat in the body, usually around the trunk area. If we eat a lot of these types of food, the mid-section weight gain is always hard to shift if unwittingly eating too much sugar. Research shows that eating too much sugar is behind the huge surge in cases of Type 2 diabetes, so not only are these low-fat foods making us fat, they are making us sick too. The low-fat food message well and truly failed us.

It's just not straightforward to define all fats as "bad." There are some fats that should be feared—the chemically derived fats, which are mainly vegetable oils, such as canola (from rapeseed), soy, sunflower, safflower and corn. These oils go through an industrial solvent extraction process, which requires a number of heating treatments and the application of chemical products (petroleum to mention one) before they are bottled and sold. Unlike butter, coconut butter and olive oils, which do not undergo these processes, vegetable oils, if being used for something like margarine, have to go through a further process called hydrogenation, which makes them solid when cooled. Do you still want to eat margarine? You can see why I'm plugging the natural fats and there are many more to be enjoyed that are essential for our health.

Why fat is actually OK

So fat was out and sugar was in, but health experts have known for years that some fats are in fact essential for good health. Eggs were let off the hook after it was discovered that even though they contained cholesterol, it was the heart healthy kind. Oily fish, such as salmon and mackerel, nuts, seeds, oils and avocados were found to contain essential fatty acids which serve multiple important health functions in the body and can only be obtained from food hence the name "essential." Every cell in the body has an outer layer that's made up of fat, so we need to consume good fats to keep these cells strong and healthy, which in turn keeps us strong and healthy.

The likes of red meat and butter are still considered bad by many. However, this is changing as more and more research reveals that even saturated fats (found in red meat and butter) are healthier than previously thought. A large Cambridge University meta-analysis (a study that looks at other studies) stated that there isn't any evidence to support the theory that saturated fat increases heart disease risk.

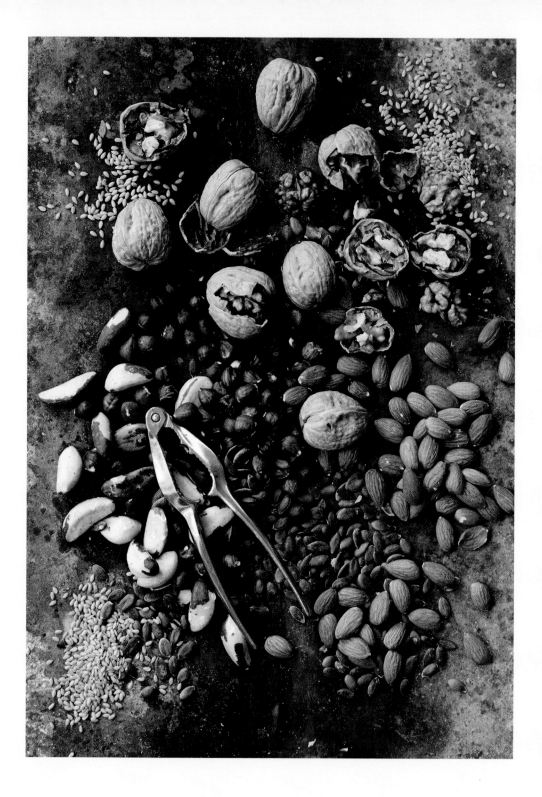

Eat. Nourish. Glow.

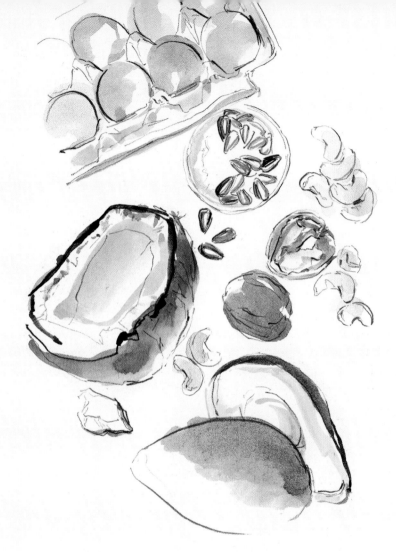

So fat isn't such a devil after all, but let's keep this in perspective—
it isn't a green light to eat all the cheese, red meat, sausages and butter you
can handle. I'm not saying ditch the margarine and slather your bread
with butter instead. I'm saying, ditch the margarine, ditch the bread and
use a little butter on some lovely vegetables. Enjoy red meat occasionally,
not daily, but make it organic and locally raised. Don't buy processed red
meats like ham, salami, sausages, ground beef and bacon that are insanely
cheap and insanely contaminated. Enjoy a small amount of good-quality

cheese if your body copes well with dairy, but make it the real type—not the processed kind that's shiny and rubbery. Be mindful about it and eat it gracefully and in moderation alongside vegetables, fruits, oils and herbs.

The beauty of fat—natural and pure fat, not the kind found in processed pies or chips—is that it tastes absolutely delicious. It is excellent to fill you up and to provide flavor in a way that low-fat/high-sugar foods just can't compete with. It also helps us reap the benefits of other foods more efficiently—a 2004 study from Iowa State University in the U.S. found that our bodies absorb more health-boosting nutrients like lycopene and betacarotene from vegetables when they are eaten together with fat, such as oil or nuts. If you eat a fat-free salad tossed in fat-free (sugar!) dressing you are negating the nutritional benefits.

I have had hundreds of clients who are fat phobic. They can reel off the calorie content of avocados and almonds and never use olive oil. They will only buy low-fat yogurts, milk and salad dressings, so it can be challenging for them to introduce natural fats into their diet. One client comes to mind who really struggled to switch her daily low-fat, berry-flavored, sweet yogurt for full-fat plain yogurt, which isn't sweet. She missed the sweet ice cream flavored yogurts so much that she started adding honey to her healthy yogurt, which just wasn't the point!

Dietary fat is known to be essential for neurological health, metabolism, joint health and, of course, skin. I can usually see if someone is deficient in essential fatty acids from their skin—flaky skin on the arms and face, a loss of plumpness to the skin—so it's time to stop worrying about the fat content of real foods—worry about the sugar content and if the food is in its real state. Avoid anything that sells itself as low fat—it's just a "Package and Promise" (see page 51) that will harm your health!

These are the fats that I encourage you to include in your diet:

Coconut butter, milk, cream, oil and meat

Olive oil

Avocados and their oil

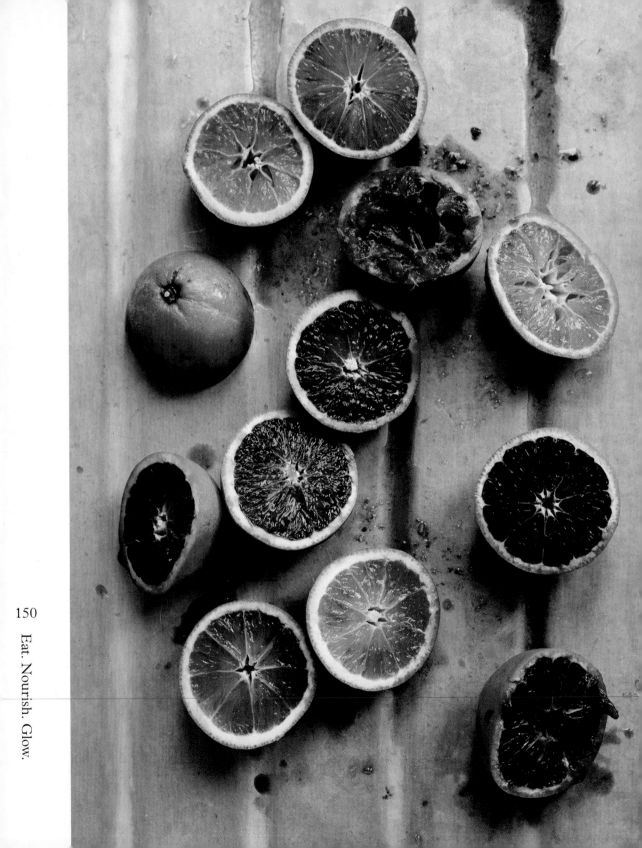

Eat. Nourish. Glow.

Nuts, seeds and their butters, milks and oils (don't cook with the oils, just use them for flavor)

Oily fish, such as salmon, mackerel, sardines and tuna

Organic butter (if you don't react to eating dairy)

Ghee

Organic red meats and poultry

The real diet villain—sugar

It's no longer new news that sugar is the real villain. This has been demonstrated by the increasing rates of obesity, Type 2 diabetes and heart disease, now known as "diabesity."

I'm not talking about the obvious sugars—it's all its forms. While we know that all fats aren't equal, in my view, sugars are! The body doesn't know the difference between a slice of bread and a pack of sweets. All carbohydrates are converted to sugar once you have eaten them so even the "healthy" forms, such as honey, fruit and whole grains are registered as "sugar" by our bodies. If you are highly active then most likely you can utilize these sugars and make energy from them, but if you are sedentary at a desk, snacking throughout the day on "sugar" means it will be converted to fat and stored around your organs and visibly around your waist. I would be a very rich woman if I had a pound for every client that told me they don't eat much sugar yet when taking a closer look at their food diary, discover they are, in fact, having a sugar-based diet in the form of carbohydrates. Regular sugar, found in cookies, and hidden sugar found in pasta sauces and low-fat yogurt, do the same thing.

"Over-vat" is a term to describe people with too much visceral fat, which is the fat that gets stored around our organs. A diet high in sugars switches the body into fat storage mode and unless we are incredibly active, we can't utilize the sugar we have consumed, so we store fat first in the liver, then in the muscles and then around our internal organs. This is visceral fat and it's one of the most dangerous types of fat you can have—linked to Type 2 diabetes, heart disease, hormonal imbalances and dementia. Visceral fat is close to the portal vein, which carries blood from the stomach area to the liver. Fatty acids and cytokines from visceral fat can enter the portal vein and go to the liver, which can lead to a fatty liver, hepatic insulin resistance and elevated triglycerides. We don't want visceral fat!

Being "over-sat" is a term to describe having an excess of subcutaneous fat. This is the squidgy soft fat you can see under your skin. Subcutaneous fat in the stomach area can increase your risk of heart disease and diabetes, just like visceral fat.

I do see many clients who are "over-vat." They are "skinny fat" in that they look slim in clothes, but are holding onto a lot of internal visceral fat. They are young and think they are getting away with a poor-quality diet, but it will catch up with them. Maybe not in the way they think—in other words, weight gain—but in the more sinister way of poor health and future diseases. We can't ignore what high sugar diets are doing to our health—ALL of us. If you are eating "healthy" sugars all day—you are in this category.

The sugar rollercoaster ride If you feel that you are addicted to sugar, rest assured you are not alone. For it is a highly addictive substance, in all its forms. The addiction is strong and studies have shown it to be more addictive than cocaine. Can we call it a drug? I always say, if you start your day on sugar, you will end your day on sugar. It's like getting on that rollercoaster. Once you have buckled in and it's started to move, you can't get off, and sugar is just the same.

This rollercoaster effect is mainly down to the role of insulin, which removes excess sugar from your bloodstream. It is pretty efficient at doing this but often can remove too much sugar, leading to what's known as a blood sugar low. These are the times when we feel hungry and a bit shaky. We need food and an apple or nuts simply won't do—we need sugar! If this is familiar to you, it's not because you are greedy or lack willpower, its because your body is hard-wired to select the fastest releasing carbohydrate within sight to stabilize your blood sugar level and get back into its comfort zone. This happens all day long—the body is a fine-tuned and incredibly efficient machine working hard all day to react and respond to the foods we eat.

Sugar also has an endorphin (which are feel-good hormones) effect on the brain and hence the comparison to cocaine. When that wears off we crave more sugar to level the feeling again. If we don't eat sugar we feel low and moody, coming down from the "high," so we reach for more. It affects us physically and emotionally—a total body highjack!

Like many other addictive substances, over time we need more and more sugar to get the same endorphin hit. The body has to produce increasing amounts of insulin to cope with the elevated sugar levels, and the more insulin that's produced, the less our cells acknowledge and respond to its presence and eventually they give up—this is Type 2 diabetes. It is entirely reversible and avoidable by managing our sugar intake.

Consume small amounts of natural sugars Don't just think of sugar as something that is making you fat—it's making you sick too. Our bodies simply aren't designed to consume such large quantities of it. It's only designed to get natural sugars from fruits and vegetables. Most of the sugar in my diet comes from fruit; I also get a little from the red wine I drink and the occasional cube of dark chocolate. My body copes fine with this, because I eat so well the rest of the time. What our bodies can't cope with is sugar at every single meal (often without realizing), which is how so many of us eat. I currently aim for 10–13 portions of fruit and vegetables a day—three portions of this are fruit, one portion per meal. The remainder will be vegetables at all three meals. In the morning I have a green juice made with cucumber, celery, fennel and spinach then I choose one piece of fruit to go in, like an apple or a portion of blueberries. Most of us do it the other way around and pile our juicers high with sugary fruit and add just one or two pieces of vegetable—often the most sugary ones like carrot and beet. Most store-bought smoothies and juices are the same, so try and pick one that's predominantly vegetables and not fruit. Of course, this advice is general—some people can cope with natural sugars better than others—use this as a guideline to become much more aware of where the sugars feature in your life.

For lunch I have a salad with different vegetables, such as lettuce, broccoli, fennel, cherry tomatoes, red onion and squash or zucchini, then I add my fruit, like sliced mango, grated pear or grilled peach—depending what's in season. For dinner I have more vegetables, followed by a bowl of anti-aging blueberries or a couple of small apricots. I never snack on fruit alone—I always have it with other foods so the sugar hit isn't so great. As I have said before, I have one source of protein at each meal so nuts, seeds, poultry, meat or fish and sometimes legumes.

Breaking the sugar cravings Because I have very little sugar in my diet I never crave it and I can't tell you how freeing that feels. Trust me, I used to be a sugar junkie! I am still horrified by how much sugar I used to eat without being aware of it. When clients tell me they are hungry for sugar I tell them to drink more water, eat more vegetables and ride out the cravings, but even if you just need to start by reducing it slowly, then that's fine too. I find that cravings reduce after a week of breaking the cycle. It will be one of the best things you ever do for your body, health, face and emotional well-being. Remember, I used to drink 10 cups of tea a day with three sugars in each, so if I can give up sugar then anybody can.

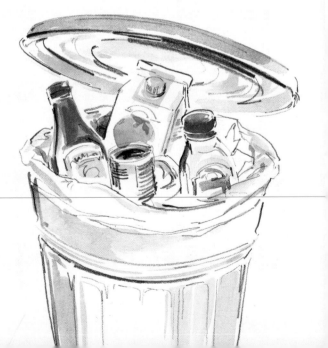

Where you will find sugar

As well as in obvious things like sweets, cookies and the white sugar added to our coffee mugs, you will also find sugar in:

Bread, rice, pasta, couscous, potatoes, polenta, oats

Breakfast cereals

Low-fat yogurts, mousses and desserts

Fruit juices, energy drinks, flavored waters, sodas and fizzy drinks

Alcohol

Muffins, croissants, bagels, baguettes and other sweet baked goods (homemade and fresh are better than the store-bought ones with long sell-by dates)

Anything with syrup, sucrose or glucose in the ingredients list

Natural sugars, such as honey, maple syrup, agave, xylitol and stevia (the brain registers them all the same)

Sauces like ketchup, brown sauce, mayonnaise and creamy salad dressings

Other salad dressings, especially low-fat ones

Artificial sweeteners

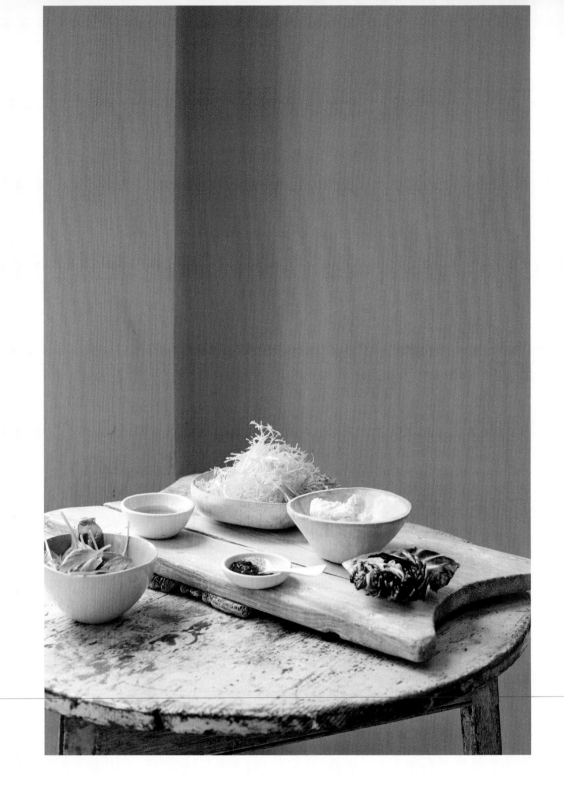

Eat. Nourish. Glow.

"Everyone has a physician inside him or her; we just have to help it in its work. The natural healing force within each one of us is the greatest force in getting well."

Hippocrates

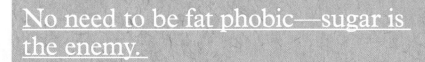

CHAPTER 6 · IN A NUTSHELL

No need to be fat phobic—sugar is the enemy.

Rewire your brain for healthy food choices / Trust your gut / Finding your natural equilibrium / Your microbiome / Happy food / Quick recipe ideas / Feel-good foods / The top seven life-force foods

<u>Why healthy food is happy food.</u>

—No. 7

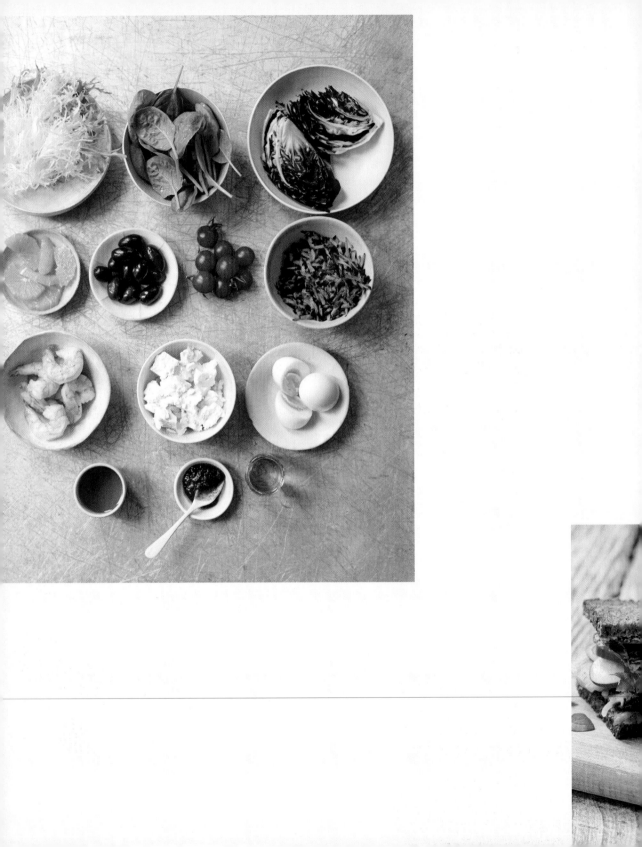

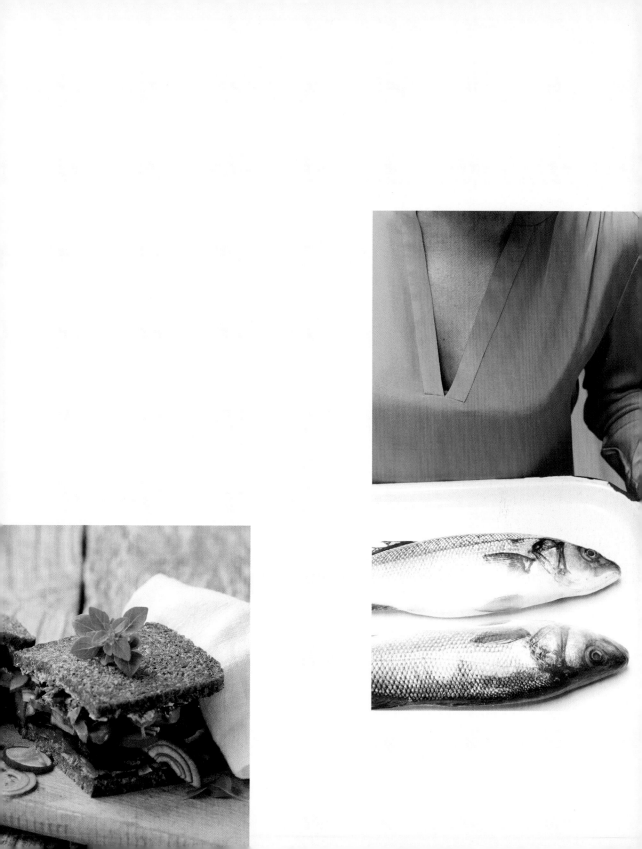

"Nutrition is not low fat. It's not low calorie. It's not being hungry and feeling deprived. It's nourishing your body with real, whole foods so that you are consistently satisfied and energized to live life to the fullest."

I once had a friend over for dinner after work. He had been working hard, not paying much attention to what he was eating and felt run down and foggy as a result. He arrived wanting pizza or starchy food. I told him I was making a salad. This didn't go down very well. Undeterred I threw some strips of chicken breast I had in the fridge into a mixing bowl. I added some sliced mango, a few large handfuls of a couple of different types of lettuce leaves, some chopped cilantro and chilies, some cooked broccoli and a sliced avocado before mixing it all together with olive oil, lime, sea salt and pepper. He begrudgingly took his first mouthful and then started to make some very positive sounds. He absolutely loved it! His mind told him he wanted pizza and that a salad would be miserable but actually all he wanted was flavor, and flavor he got. He had no idea that healthy food could be tasty and satisfying. Much to my frustration, healthy food just can't seem to escape the "drab" reputation. I regularly see clients who arrive and state almost immediately that they won't eat bird food! I assure them that neither will I. They usually find my approach quite refreshing when I tell them how much I love food, how much I celebrate and enjoy it and that I never go hungry or deprived. It's usually a big relief as they arrive expecting to be put "on a diet" and are mentally preparing themselves for people to feel sorry for them or challenge them. There's such a stigma attached to eating well and the idea that healthy food is boring, tasteless and for hippies! I hope you have found from reading the rest of this book that it's possible to have a different attitude and to change preconceived ideas about how to be healthy.

Naturally I blame the diet industry. Anyone wanting to lose weight has, up until now, been led to believe that you need to be hungry and drink revolting shakes, plastic microwave meals or dull salads to get in shape. We know that deprivation leads to misery, dull food AND feeling hungry—who can stick with that? What cost does this way of eating and thinking have on our health? Our brains? Our digestive system?

There are so many people walking around feeling unhappy about their weight or their health. They are eating "comfort" foods to make them feel happy, but those foods keep them overweight and ill and so the cycle continues. They then seek advice to make changes and the fear of eating differently—fresh foods like salads, vegetables and fruit—produces much rolling of the eyeballs. I have seen it hundreds of times. It's a tough cycle to break, but the ramifications of just one change can be enormous and enough to wire the brain for a different, happy, more positive state, just from enjoying a healthy plate of food. We can choose to retrain our taste buds and the foods we "think" we enjoy.

Anecdotally, I see that a person can experience change in their health when making dietary improvements—I have noted clients with better sleep, more comfortable digestion, clearer minds, brighter moods, relief from aching joints, glowing skin, reduction of headaches, reduction of eczema and psoriasis—in just seven days. That's just the start.

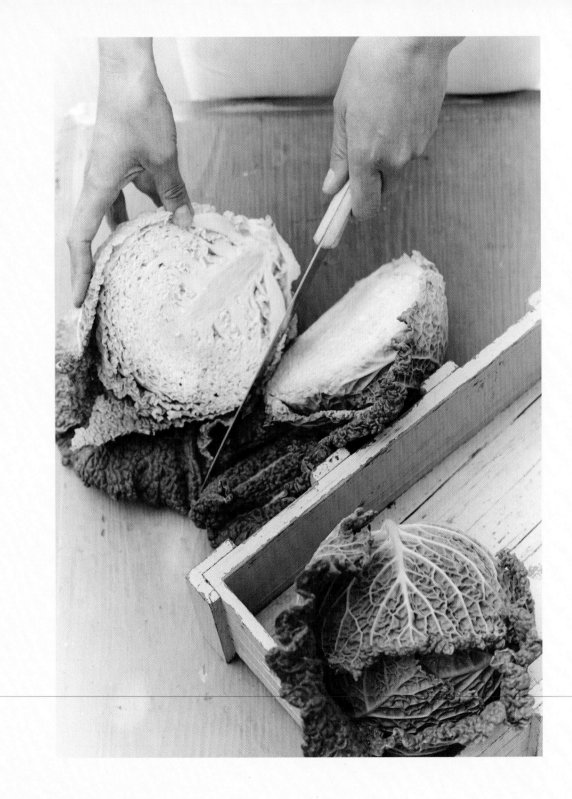

Eat. Nourish. Glow.

"Happiness is homemade."

Trust your gut

This leads me to the actual process of eating. Our digestive system is such a magnificent and fine-tuned machine. The very process of digestion begins with the sights, sounds, smells and even thoughts of food. The brain responds to these senses by signaling the release of digestive juices in our saliva and stomach. So even before your first bite, the digestive process has begun. Let's talk about this bite. We don't have teeth in our stomach, only in our mouth and their function is one of the most important stages of digestion. The aim is to chew thoroughly, to allow the food to be well mixed with the saliva so that when the broken down food enters the stomach the next stage of digestion can begin. In the stomach we only have muscle and a combination of digestive juices, which continue to break the food down into a soup consistency. So if you inhaled your food instead of chewing it, you are making tough work for your stomach and incomplete digestion is likely to occur, which can create a feeding ground for bad bacteria. Now you may not think that this has anything to do with happiness, but let me assure you it does. Our digestive system and our brains are interconnected. We have our central nervous system (brain and spinal cord) and our enteric nervous system (gastrointestinal tract). Research has long proven that the brain sends signals to our guts, but more recently it has been discovered that this also works in reverse—yes our gut communicates with our brain, in fact more than the brain does to our gut. So while you may be aware that you get butterflies in your tummy if nervous, you may not be aware that you can suffer anxiety or depression if there are problems in your gut. There is also a wealth of evidence linking gastrointestinal involvement with neurological disease. What sort of messages do you think your gut is sending to your brain?

Enter the microbiome. We have our very own tiny ecosystem, over a trillion microorganisms, our own community of bacteria inside us. These bacteria reside in our guts, brain, skin, lungs, mouth and nasal passage and far outnumber our cells, making us more bacteria than cellular! But not all bacteria need to be put on the naughty step. We are meant to have a perfect equilibrium of the good and the bad. The problem is that a poor lifestyle and diet, riddled with stress, eating in a hurry and not chewing, taking copious amounts of antibiotics, eating chemically enhanced and poor quality food, using antibacterial soaps, eating non-organic vegetables and meat is literally like feeding the opposition and helping them to grow strong inside us. Eating this way encourages war within your very own community. Studies have found that the balance of the gut bacteria can also contribute toward obesity, immune function, learning difficulties and autism and diabetes. It's an area that is now getting much attention and a lot more research.

We must think outside the box when it comes to which foods we think make us happy and which don't. We do have two brains and both need to be nurtured and nourished.

Happy food

Despite choosing healthy foods I still love comforting foods. The old favorites of pasta, pies, pizza and fries are still doable in healthier ways (see the recipes on pages 220–59). I love to take the unhealthy foods from cookbooks and switch the ingredients to make a healthier, healing and happier version; it's one of the best parts of my job. I also love the challenge of helping a client to try new foods, and recreate their favorite meals so that they will feel great and get excited about eating in a new way. I remember getting a call from a client when he realized that he does in fact like avocados—it was a great day for me! Here are some favorite "comfort foods" I have created over the years . . .

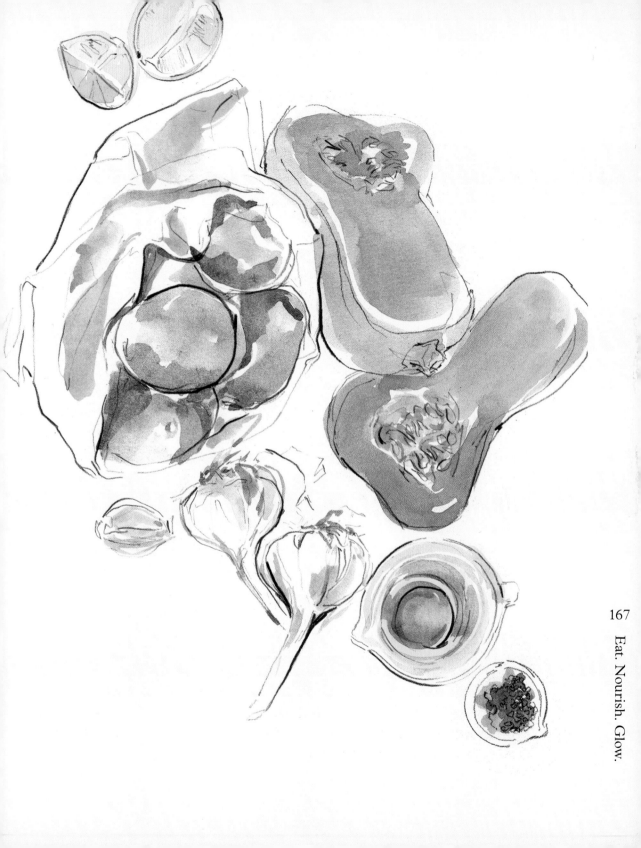

Eat. Nourish. Glow.

Quick lunchtime omelet

Sauté some chopped onions and peppers in a pan with a little coconut oil and a pinch of paprika. Remove from the pan and set aside. Beat two eggs and pour into the pan. Cook, moving the pan regularly to prevent the egg from sticking. Once solidified and almost cooked, sprinkle the onions and peppers on top then fold the omelet in half and heat until the egg is cooked through. Top with some sliced avocado and a sprinkle of chopped fresh chilies.

Chicken arrabiata

One of my favorite foods used to be penne arrabiata, which is pasta in a spicy sauce made with tomatoes, garlic and chilies. This is my version:

Put a spoonful of coconut oil in a pan and add chopped onion, chopped garlic and a fresh chilies (I have these pre-chopped in the freezer). Throw in a handful of fresh cherry tomatoes, some tomato puree and two chicken breasts. Stir, turn the heat down and cover with a lid. Leave to steam/poach for 20 minutes, or until the chicken is cooked through. The chicken remains tender and the sauce is rich and flavorful. It's a lazy but delicious dish. I serve it with a large green salad and I love that there is little washing up to do afterward. It's perfect for when the weather is cold and you crave something warm and comforting.

Burgers don't need to be in a bun, nor do they need to be filled with breadcrumbs, dripping in cheese or burned on a barbecue. I make turkey burgers with sun-dried tomatoes and fresh herbs and wrap them in crunchy lettuce leaves with a dollop of herby mayo (see below), and it's far better than any fast-food chain burger (yes I used to eat those!). You can do the same with lamb, beef or chicken. They are so simple to make—just mix with a sautéed onion and some herbs. I often make up large batches and store a few in the freezer for lazy days.

◖ Homemade herby "mayonnaise"

Soak a large handful of cashews overnight in water. The next day, drain the cashews and pop them in a blender with a little Himalayan pink sea salt, some fresh lemon juice, garlic and any herbs you like and blend. If it's a little too thick add small amounts of water until it has a mayonnaise-like consistency. I enjoy this mayo spread on buckwheat toast with sliced cucumber or avocado. If you like spicy food, give your mayo a kick with some fresh chilies and lime juice.

Need a quick dessert for friends coming to dinner? Place some coconut yogurt in a bowl and sprinkle some fresh berries on top.

—Tip

I use my food processor with the slicing option to pre-chop onions, garlic, chilies and fresh herbs. I divide them up into small batches, then put them in paper bags and keep them in the freezer. This means I have a constant supply of pre-chopped flavors ready to use when I'm in a hurry to prepare a meal.

—Tip

I also use my food processor to mix up different flavorings, for example an Asian mix of chopped chilies, garlic, cilantro, turmeric and ginger or onion, garlic and ginger or rosemary, thyme, parsley, lemon zest and garlic, which can be added to sautéed vegetables for stir-fries or marinades for meat or fish. You can also freeze these in ice-cube trays with olive oil or melted coconut butter to add quick flavor to a dish.

Feel-good foods

Several studies have found that eating certain foods really does make us happier. Researchers in New Zealand recently found that study participants who ate more vegetables and fruit reported feeling calmer and happier soon after eating them—this could be due to an improved blood sugar response but also due to the bacteria—change can occur within one day. It's not just fruits and vegetables that boost your mood, it's eating well in general. By that I mean eating a good range of fruits, vegetables, meat or non-meat protein sources, seeds, nuts, oils and herbs and steering clear of processed foods. Think of processed foods as empty short-term energy and real foods as a life force. Here are some that are particularly good:

Fermented foods: These are one of the most fantastic ways to supply beneficial bacteria to your digestive system and include fermented vegetables, fermented milk such as kefir and kombucha, a fermented tea. Fermenting is an ancient way to preserve foods. Probably the most widely available now are sauerkraut or cabbage, but pretty much any vegetable can be fermented if you do it yourself. If you buy it ready made make sure you are not buying a pasteurized version.

Healthy fats: These include coconut oil, avocados, organic and free range eggs, wild salmon, olive oil, olives, milk and butter. They are well regarded as playing an important role in brain health.

Dark green leafy vegetables: These vegetables contain folate, which studies have found may reduce the symptoms of depression because folate is used by the brain to produce feel-good hormones like serotonin and dopamine. There are so many excellent sources to choose from including spinach, kale, chard, broccoli and cabbage.

Oily fish: Natural sources of polyunsaturated fatty acids are present in oily fish, which help to improve brain function and mood control.

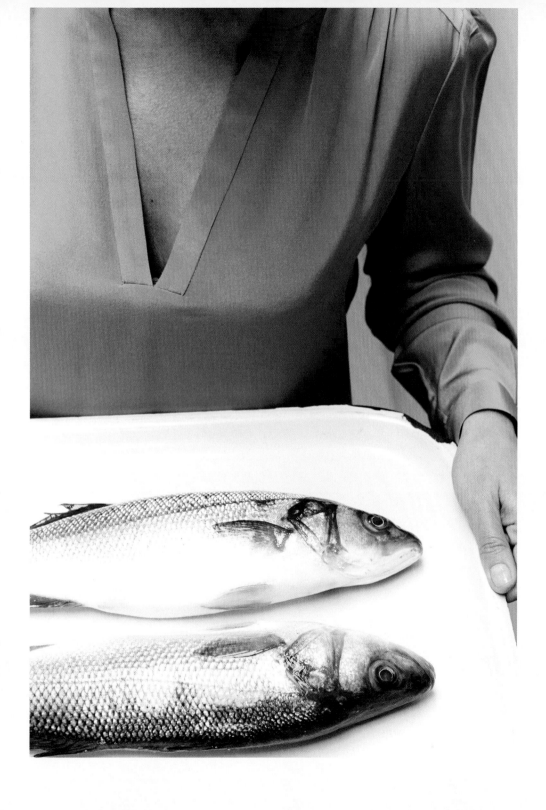

Eat. Nourish. Glow.

There is an established link between low levels of omega-3 fatty acids (found in oily fish and some nuts) and depression. The best oily fish are salmon, tuna, mackerel, herring and sardines. However, eating fish is now somewhat controversial because of overfishing and so we ideally want to aim to eat the most sustainable fish, which means locally sourced. Try to be conscious and check where the fish you buy has come from.

Broccoli and cauliflower: These contain choline, a B vitamin essential for brain development and considered to boost brain function. Eggs and meat are also sources of choline.

Walnuts: These nuts are an excellent source of omega-3 essential fatty acids known to boost brain function.

Blueberries: These contain antioxidants that are regarded to be brain protective and can reduce oxidative stress.

172

173

Our happiness can directly be affected by
the food choices we make, on many levels.

Are you dehydrated? /
Hydration and your digestive
health / Cut down on caffeine /
Alcohol / Healthy hydration /
Which water to drink? /
Retrain your taste buds and
appreciate flavor / How
we can hydrate with food /
Juicing

Are you eating instead of drinking?

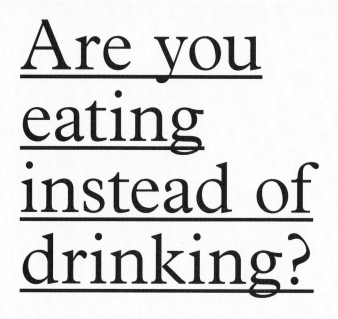

—No. 8

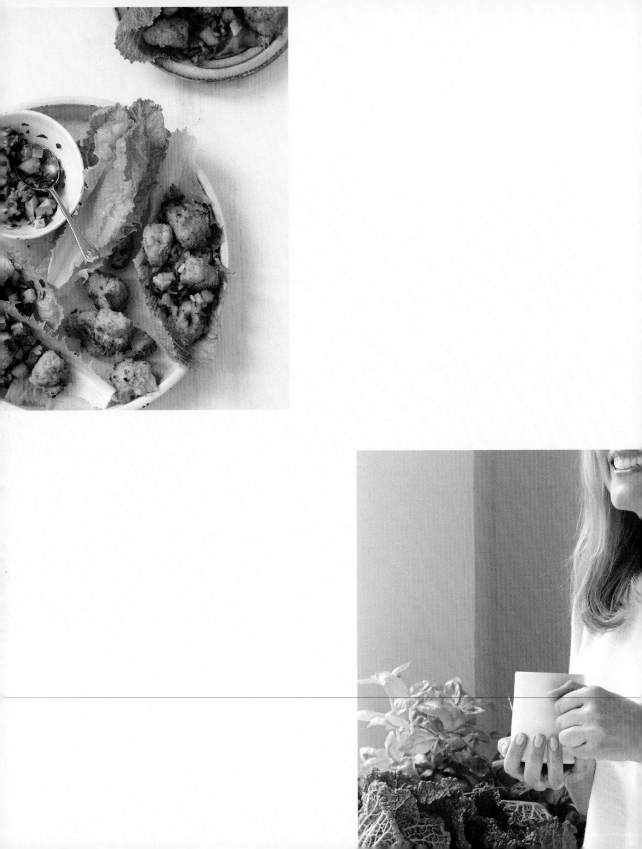

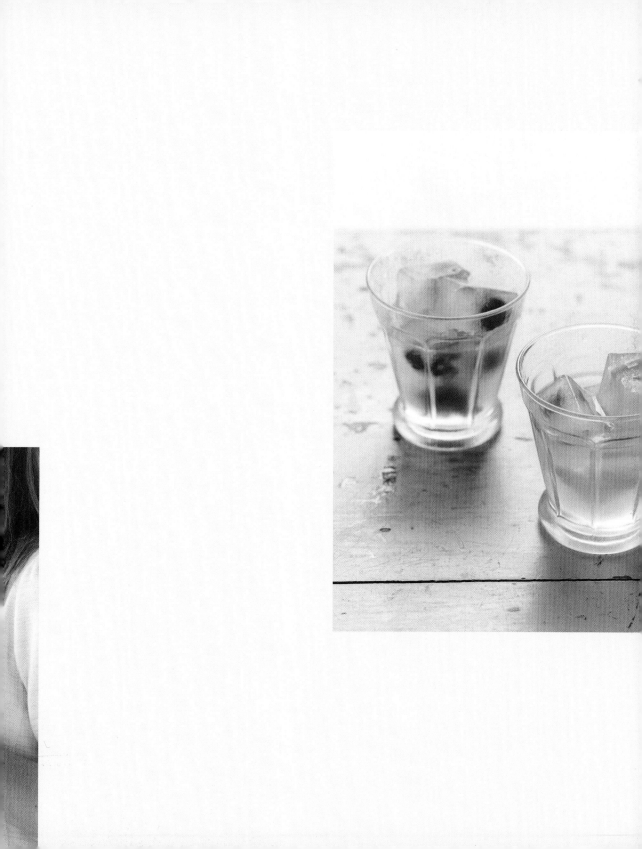

> "Change occurs when the pain of remaining the same is greater than the pain of changing.'

It is well known that water is essential for our survival. We are each made up of roughly 60 percent water and while we can survive for months without food, we can only live for a few days without water. Our body loses water daily through sweat, breath and urine so we must replenish it every day. Yet the guidelines for how much we should drink are unclear and the standard "eight glasses a day" is not a credible or researched recommendation. We do need water but how much is up to each individual. What I am more concerned about is the types of hydration that are on offer and regularly consumed in place of pure water, and the impact they can have on how we look, feel and eat.

I used to be incredibly dehydrated. I didn't know it at the time but looking back I can see just how much my lack of hydration was feeding into my declining health. I drank sweet tea from a very young age and the habit continued right up until my early twenties—from the moment I woke up to the time I went to bed I was drinking tea with three added sugars. I would get headaches if I didn't drink it and whenever I felt tired or hungry during the day I would have another cup. The rest of my diet was far from perfect but it was my sweet tea addiction that really dictated how I felt and what I ate—no wonder I was constipated, had acne, headaches, felt exhausted and couldn't concentrate for long! My blood sugar was on a constant rollercoaster from all the caffeine and sugar, and I was exhausted and always hungry for carbs and sugar! I wasn't really hungry. I was dehydrated. If I had been able to be more mindful back then I would have realized what an addictive habit I was in and that I wasn't listening to my body and its request for water.

I always ask my clients "how do you hydrate?" They answer fruit juice, tea, coffee, sodas, alcohol—very rarely does pure water feature. I think the humble water has been replaced by our quest for flavor and the rise of vitamin waters and fruit juices has dumbed us and our taste buds down just a little too much. What is key to understand is that every other form of liquid will affect our blood sugar level and raise insulin—every single one. So maybe they might provide a little replenishment of water but they will also be dumping insulin and inflammation at the same time.

That is not to say that the odd cup of tea, coffee, wine or fruit juice can't be enjoyed from time to time, but the sodas, sports drinks, fruit juices and artificial sweetened drinks have to go. Yes even the fancy, healthy looking ones. The expensive baby pink lemonades in glass bottles; the lovely looking pastel colored "fruit waters"; those deliciously described cordials that have pretty labels on the bottle; even the fruit smoothies— they are all just liquid sugar.

Our needs for water are individual. Exercise, temperature and working conditions can alter a person's needs. The best indicators are listening to your body—symptoms such as headaches, low energy, lack of concentration, dry skin and constipation, and the best guidelines are thirst and the color of your urine, which should be a pale yellow (unless you have been taking supplements with B vitamins, which can change the color to a dark yellow). Now that I am in tune with my body, I know exactly how much water I need to drink to make me feel and look my best. I don't believe that water should be forced or drunk in large quantities at one time, but instead, something that should be consistent throughout the day. Certainly an excess of water is not at all advisable, so if you forget to drink water during the day, don't go home and drink 2 quarts at once. It's not about checking off a certain quantity each day. I believe it's about making it your drink of choice and replacing all of the other forms of drinks that are commercially available. As a structure for clients to follow I suggest a glass every couple of hours during the waking day.

What about tea and coffee?

I know these are a passionate staple in most of our lives and naturally clients are always fearful that I will take them away. I won't. As a reformed caffeine addict, I get it! I did, however, have to go through a tough period reducing and even eliminating it for a period while I got my health back on track, and once out the other side it was great. It's a nice place to be when not dependent on them but able to still enjoy them. I'm relaxed about caffeine. There is a place for it in a healthy diet, depending on the health of the individual of course. Some people are incredibly sensitive to caffeine and those who are enduring high levels of stress may be best without it—excess adrenaline is not a long-term productive state. But for those who aren't too stressed, fatigued or sensitive to it, then one cup of pure, unadulterated (no sugar, sweeteners or milk), organic, good-quality caffeine per day is not such a bad thing. It's the overuse of it that is to be avoided.

Starting your day on pure caffeine is not ideal. First, we sweat a lot when we sleep so when we wake up our bodies need hydration. Tea and coffee are simply not a good enough form of hydration to do this job, and as natural diuretics, they are considered by some to counteract hydration. Second, if you start your day with caffeine then you will start yourself off on a bad blood sugar cycle. So have water first, then your breakfast, then your caffeine. This is general advice—if you are super-healthy and fit and do intermittent fasting then you already know how to listen to your body.

There are, however, quite a few reported benefits to caffeine. It has been found to lift mood, contains health-boosting antioxidants, improves athletic performance before a workout and boosts concentration and alertness. But as with food, there is caffeine and then there is real caffeine, particularly in the case of coffee! You may scoff at the idea of spending money on good coffee, but how much are you spending per day on poor-quality cappuccinos and lattes from the café near work? Organic is naturally the best coffee to opt for.

There are also many studies reporting benefits of tea. Black tea is considered to reduce stress levels; like coffee it contains antioxidants and some studies suggest it can protect heart health. So yes, tea can be part of a healthy diet as long as it's drunk in moderation (due to the caffeine it contains) and you don't add lots of sugar and milk to it. If, like I used to be, you are a total tea junkie who has sugar in their tea then start slowly.

When I first saw a nutritional therapist and she told me I needed to cut right back on tea I thought she was crazy. How on earth was I supposed to do that when it was such a huge part of my life? But I have managed it and you can too. Start by gradually reducing the amount of sugar and milk you have. If you have three sugars, go down to two. After a week you won't notice the difference. Then reduce it to one sugar, before giving it up altogether. Begin to reduce the milk or swap it for a healthier substitute like almond or coconut milk, and at the same time gradually reduce the number of cups you have throughout the day. I did this until I was down to two cups a day, then I switched to Earl Grey tea, which is naturally very sweet so I didn't need any sugar or milk. Eventually I gave it up altogether. Again, opt for organic or loose leaf tea as regular tea bags contain chemicals and flavorings. READ LABELS!

I will admit that coffee is a new feature in my life and I'm having to manage it! I only had it for the first time a year ago when I was in California and was offered a supremely "healthy" version blended with coconut butter. It was delicious and I was instantly hooked! This is a new love but I'm keeping it clean and only drinking one per day. My body is not too clean to go down any slippery slope with caffeine again.

Our caffeine habits are also very much a daily ritual. Often it's the ritual that we miss more than the actual substance. Tea—and more recently coffee—is such a huge part of our culture. For me, growing up I learned to associate a "nice cup of tea" with getting home after a long day, or catching up with a friend, or the answer to all of life's troubles. "I'll put the kettle on" is often a solution to everything in Britain. I still do it, but I just drink hot water instead. It has the same effect once I allowed my brain to accept the change!

Hydration and your digestive health

It's common for people to rely on tea or coffee in the morning to encourage a bowel movement. First, I advise them to drink more water, not coffee or tea. When we are dehydrated, our body absorbs water from our stool, which then makes the stool harder and dehydrated and hence less easy to move along the digestive tract. Lubricating the stool is

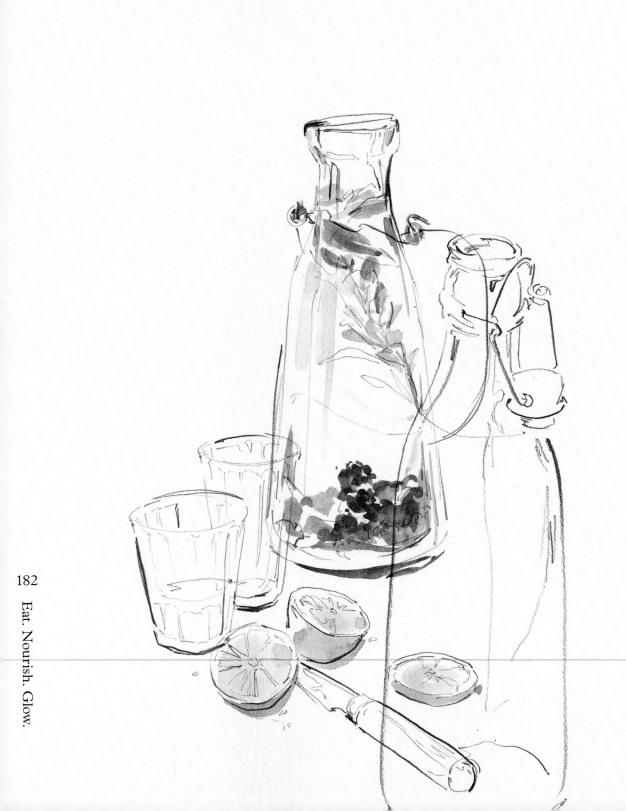

Eat. Nourish. Glow.

essential. Good fats can also help —oily fish, avocados and nuts, seeds and their oils and butters. And "heed the call." Don't ever put it off or wait until you get home as this can make constipation worse and train the bowels to become lazy. Always go when you feel the need to go. A lot of women—and some men, although I find it's more common among women—find this difficult, as they need to be in a safe and private place to feel comfortable enough to go to the bathroom. We are always rushing out the door to work at the very time we need to go, but it must be made a priority and a time set aside. If you drink a large glass of warm water when you wake up, stay hydrated the rest of the time, eat a diet full of vegetables and good fats and avoid foods that you know don't agree with you, then your digestion should really improve and not be so dependent on caffeine.

Alcohol

There are numerous studies showing that alcohol consumption, particularly red wine, can have some health benefits, but this is, of course, moderate drinking and dependent on what and how we drink. We all know that excessive consumption of alcohol can have devastating effects on both our physical and mental health from excess weight, reduced liver function, hormonal imbalance, brain damage and breast cancer to name a few links. It's also incredibly dehydrating, so naturally, I don't encourage it as your main source of hydration! It's common to drink alcohol when, in fact, we are thirsty, just as we can turn to food, so my rule of thumb is to always have a glass of water before drinking or eating, and when drinking alcohol, make it good quality (not cheap booze loaded with sugary sodas thanks!) and make sure that you drink water with it. A quick note on wine—there are now many natural wines available that are produced using traditional methods which means with minimal interference, free from pesticides, commercial yeasts and low or no sulphites. This is my wine of choice when I do drink.

"What you think about, you bring about."

Healthy hydration

I don't drink a huge variety of drinks—just filtered water, one cup of coffee, green juice or smoothie and occasionally red wine, mostly on weekends. That's it. I never drink fruit, flavored or fizzy drinks. I do, however, occasionally use coconut water in my green smoothie or green juice—it's great to take the edge off earthy greens. I start my day with two large glasses of warm water, which has been boiled then left to cool down. Sometimes I add 1 teaspoon of apple cider vinegar or some lemon slices to it, but often I just enjoy it on its own. It's amazing how it wakes me up and I don't crave caffeine in the same way I used to. I don't have a certain amount of water that I aim to drink each day nor do I gulp it down, I sip it slowly throughout the day, as and when I need.

Which water to drink?

It can get very confusing to know which is the right water to drink. From environmental concerns of bottled water to the chemicals in tap water, it can be hard to know how to safely hydrate, and we all have a right to clean water. Here's the lowdown:

Tap water

While it may be the cheapest and most convenient, tap water unfortunately also contains a host of toxic substances. These substances differ depending where you live.

Plastic bottled water

This may be the next most widely available and convenient option, but the plastic bottles contain a chemical called Bisphenol A or BPA, which is known to be a hormone disrupter and hence may have implications in prostate and breast cancer, weight issues, early puberty and immune health. It is also suggested that some bottled water is just tap water! Of course there is also the environmental damage that plastic bottles are causing from the toxic chemicals released into the environment when the plastic is made, to the landfills and our oceans filled with them. I try to take my own water with me when out traveling, and if I do buy bottled water I try to get glass bottles where I can.

Filtered

There are now numerous filters available to clean out some of the nasties in our tap water. This is currently the best option that I know of for getting the cleanest water, but none are able to clean up 100 percent of our water. I use a reverse osmosis filter which takes out most of the chemicals and pollutants, but it does also take out the minerals so I ensure that I add Himalayan pink salt (see page 56) to my diet to counteract this.

Coconut water

Coconut water has become very trendy now and there are health benefits to it—it contains some electrolytes, but it's not a health tonic as some press suggests. It's an excellent alternative to water for those who find water too bland, so I will often recommend it for this reason, but it still contains fruit sugars—especially if you are opting for the flavored ones, which I don't advise. I'm certain that we will see a lot more highjacked coconut waters popping up on supermarket shelves over the next few years and I doubt they will be the healthy kinds, so beware of the fads and stick with unpasturized, unflavored, 100 percent pure coconut water.

Flavor

As I have said throughout this book, it is possible to re-train our taste buds and not be dependent on a need for sugar or flavor, so I also encourage this with water. However, if you really struggle to drink it "straight" then here are a few healthy ways to hydrate your water with added natural flavor:

Fruit and herbs

If you find water boring you can add healthy flavors to it like lemon, cucumber, orange or apple slices or fresh herbs like mint and basil. Sometimes I add a green tea bag and a slice of lemon to a large jug of cold water and sip that throughout the day. Herbal teas are equally a great way of keeping your water levels topped up. Fruit teas aren't as good, due to the fructose (fruit sugar) content. Be wary of the caffeine content also—healthy teas like green and white tea still contain caffeine so don't drink them to excess and preferably with meals and not in between. Here are a few fruit, herb and chilled tea combinations I enjoy:

Infused water & ice cubes

Watermelon and rosemary
Grape and anise
Cucumber and mint
Blueberry and vanilla pod
Apple and rose
Orange and rosemary
Lime and basil
Ginger and mango
Kiwi and lime
Raspberry and mint
Pineapple and sage
Chai, rooibos and orange
Green tea and elderflower
Matcha and pomegranate
Blueberry and lemon balm

Fruit & herb ice cubes

These are a fun way to liven up water and make it more fun, flavored and colorful. Kids love these. I like to use coconut water but they work well with filtered water too. You can use whole berries or citrus fruits cut into small quarters, depending on the size of your ice-cube trays. Ultimately, just be creative and have fun—they can't go wrong!
I also freeze cooled herbal teas—chai, rooibos or green tea are particularly good added to water.

Here are a few of my favorite combinations:

Lime and basil
Mango and mint
Orange and rosemary
Raspberry and basil
Cucumber and mint

All these combinations work well with each other so mix them up and try out different blends. Thin strips of fresh ginger made with a vegetable peeler or star anise, cinnamon or vanilla are other great flavorings to include. There are endless possibilities to make your water a little more interesting to keep you hydrated during the day.
You can make popsicles this way too.

Coconut water ice cubes

How to make them: Place your fruit slice or herb or combination of choice into a clean ice-cube tray, then fill with coconut or pure water and freeze. These are great to add to a jar of water or individual glasses.

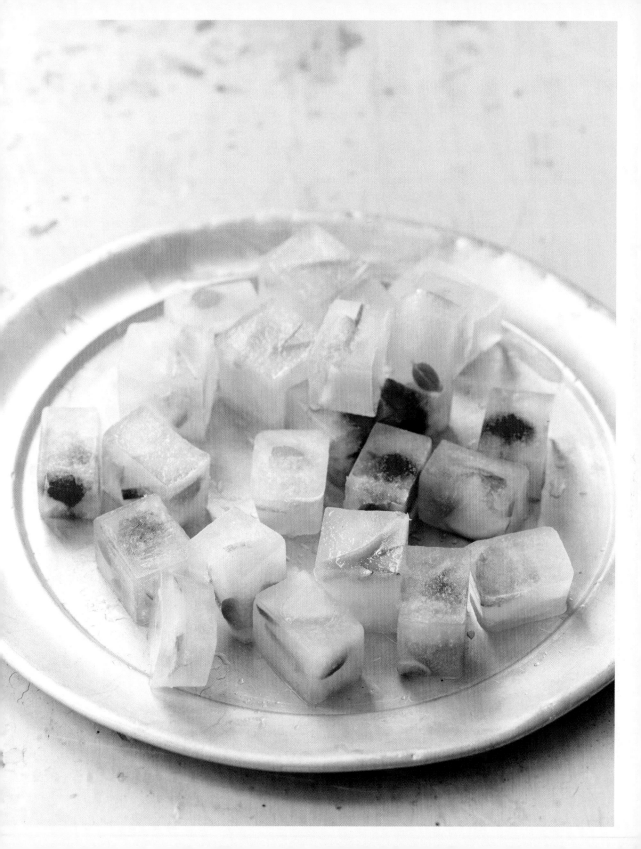

How we can hydrate with food

Other than pure, clean water, we can also hydrate with some foods, which can be of great benefit to our skin and health, too. All fruits and vegetables contain some water, and juicing and blending can be a great way to pack in nutrients as well as to hydrate. I am not a fan of juice cleansing—for healthy meals we need proteins and fats so I think that juices are a great addition, but not a replacement for your three meals a day, and a great way to give radiance, energy and optimize your health. Make sure you only use organic vegetables and fruit when juicing or blending otherwise you are just drinking juiced or blended chemicals—not so appealing!

—A note on juicing

I think that the best juicer is the one that you actually use. There are many that are complicated and hard work to clean which may put you off using them altogether! The best ones are ones that cold press. This means that they don't use heat to separate the juice from the fiber, which can destroy some of the enzymes of the fruit and vegetables and oxidize the nutrients. A cold-pressed juice gets pressed, it's slower to make but certainly produces a more nutritious end result.

Here are two of my regulars:

🥣 Rainbow juice

1 beet, peeled and chopped
4 rainbow chard leaves (or spinach)
1 orange, peeled
½-in cube of fresh ginger, peeled
Juice of ½ lemon
½ cucumber

Juice and drink.

Green smoothie

½ cucumber
A small handful of spinach
1 avocado, peeled and pitted
8 fresh mint leaves
Juice of 1 lemon
2 teaspoons chia seeds
8 oz. coconut water

Blend until smooth then drink.

CHAPTER 8 · IN A NUTSHELL

Don't drink your sugar, keep hydrated instead of overeating, and drink water regularly throughout the day.

Start with proper nutrition and you may not need to supplement / You get what you pay for—buy the best you can afford / Probiotics / Vitamin D_3 / Essential fatty acids—why they are important and where to find them

Do you need supplements?

—No. 9

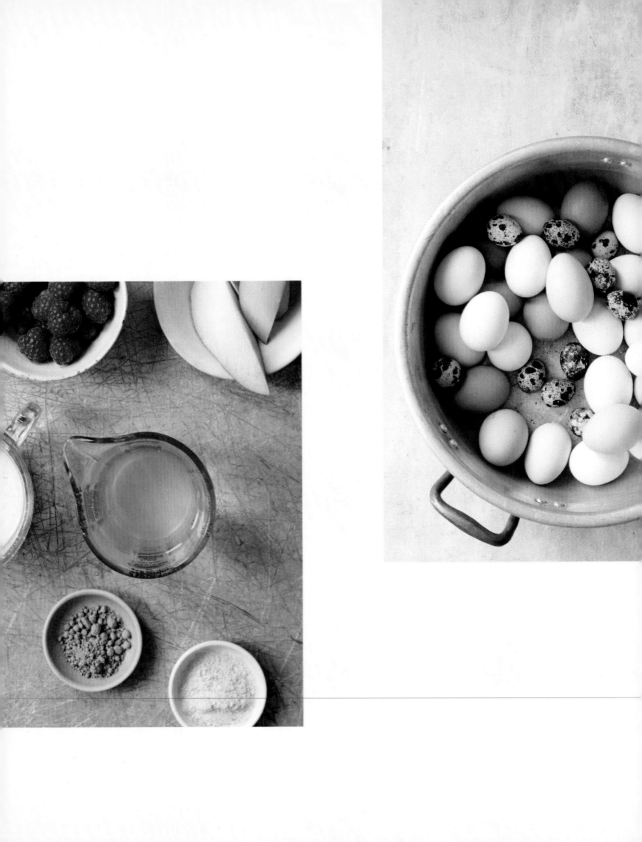

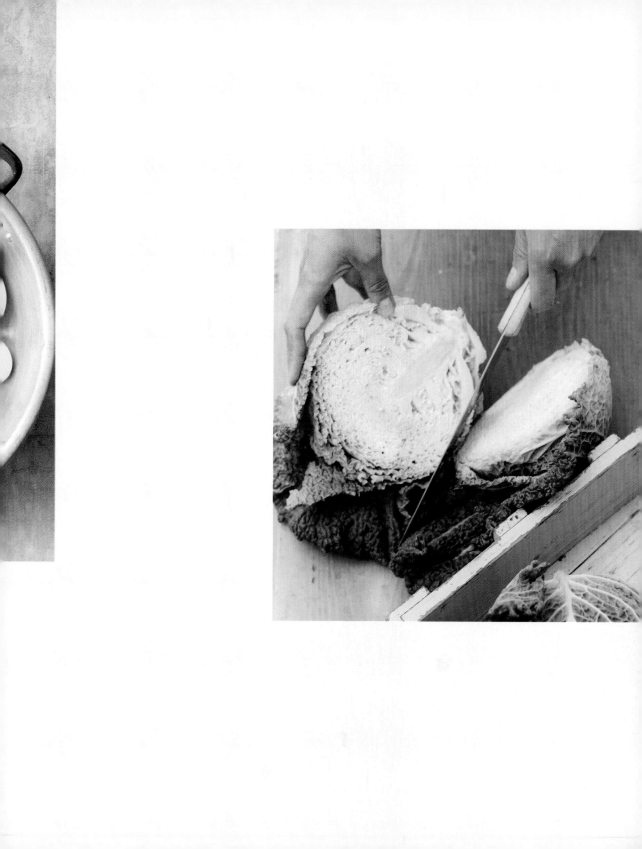

> # "Most people have no idea how good their body is designed to feel."

Kevin Trudeau

The most common question a nutritional therapist is asked is "what supplements should I take?" So many people are more inclined to pop a pill than change their diet and will happily spend money on them in the hope of quick fixes or miracle cures. They have read in a magazine or heard from friends about a certain supplement being good for improving energy levels or increasing fat burning, or something similar, so have bought the supplement, and either take it a few times before forgetting about it or take it mindlessly every day without really knowing if it's doing them any good.

It's not unusual for clients to arrive with bagfuls of supplements. Some are out of date, not very good quality, or not at all relevant to their health. Or they have been to multiple practitioners and been advised to take heaps of different supplements, too many for them and so they give up and end up back at square one. There's a sense of utter bewilderment and confusion surrounding supplements. Many people don't know if they need them, how to take them or what to take. It's a minefield, and most are getting it very wrong.

Like so much else to do with health and diet, I find there's a lot of "mindlessness" around supplements. People buy them and take them without giving much thought. They want to be healthy and they are trying their best, but they have so many other things to think about and juggle.

Just like in the food industry, there's a lot of expensive marketing and false promises going on in the supplement industry. There are also a lot of cheaply produced and processed supplements that have been heavily marketed to look healthier than they actually are. Yes, it's more "Packages and Promises."

I'm not here to tell you what supplements to take—I couldn't possibly know without seeing you in person, finding out about your diet and lifestyle and running the appropriate blood tests. Nutritional therapy is about personalized nutrition targeted toward each individual's needs and to complement a healthy lifestyle, which manages stress, gets adequate sleep and a natural diet. When I'm asked to give quotes or list my favorite supplements I always do so with caution because I don't want to add to the confusion or the fads. Ideally, supplements that are recommended to you by a healthcare practitioner will most likely be of pharmaceutical grade and from respected companies. They will understand how to use them safely and optimally in order for them to be of benefit to your individual needs.

Your health must start with your nutrition, and with real food. Absolutely no supplement can replace the benefits of a healthy lifestyle. Many people will challenge me saying that they want to get all their nutrients purely from a good diet and I agree to a certain point. I'm not a pill pusher and I would far rather a client concentrate on getting their diet right before we bring in supplements, but as you have discovered from reading this book, having a healthy diet isn't always so easy. It takes effort and is dependent on where our food is sourced, how it's grown, cooked and, of course what we select to eat. For someone who is healthy, symptom free and eating a really clean diet, then perhaps they don't need to focus heavily on supplements, but I still believe that supplements can play a supportive and preventative role in our health, and can be of benefit to everyone, healthy or not. I don't blindly suggest supplements—I conduct many functional tests to find out what's going on with that client and what their needs are first. The truth is, for those with poor health or those who wish to support their health, the right supplements can really make a difference. I honestly couldn't have helped so many clients (or myself) get back on track with their health without the use of supplements. They are so much more than vitamin C. If used correctly, safely and appropriately they can be the addition to a healthy diet that can shift our health back into balance. Don't go and self-prescribe—invest in an appointment with a qualified nutritional therapist and learn what you need, the dosage, when and for how long and how much to take. It will save you money in the long run as you will stop buying all of the random supplements that end up in the back of the cupboard unused.

I am not going to tell you what my favorites are as there are hundreds for different uses, at different times, for different conditions, and that is the targeted nutrition that I practice, through the lens of the functional medicine principles. But I will give you some general guidance for those of you who are not able to see a nutritional therapist or functional medical practitioner to help clarify some of the confusion around supplements and take the supplements that I feel everyone can benefit from.

You get what you pay for

If you are going to take supplements then buy the best ones you can afford. If you are paying very little money for your supplements it's almost certainly because there are very few nutrients. Cheaply produced supplements are often bulked up with fillers that provide nothing in the way of health and are simply passed through the body. They aren't always created in a form that's available for the human body to utilize efficiently. In short, if you are going to take supplements it's far better to buy the absolute best and take them for a short amount of time, rather than buy cheap ones and take them every day for years. A supermarket or generic supplement is certainly something that I would avoid.

Probiotics

As I discussed in Chapter Seven, good digestion is the cornerstone of good health and supporting our internal bacterial community has been shown to be of major importance to our well-being. The majority of our immune system resides in our gut—it's the headquarters of the whole system, but that's just the start. Research is relatively new in this area, but studies are suggesting that we are basically humans living in a bacterial body, and that these bacteria can impact our entire health. Due to our modern way of living, eating and the overuse of antibiotics we are killing a lot of the beneficial bacteria that we need to thrive.

So what probiotic to buy?

When I say "good quality" I mean the type that costs more money and has to be kept in the fridge. Unfortunately not all probiotics are what they seem. Read the labels and buy one that offers "billions" not "millions" of bacteria. The better the quality, the more live and viable they are and hence able to take up residence in our guts, as they are made to withstand the very acidic environment of our stomachs. The poorer quality, cheaper ones simply don't survive the digestive process.

—One last tip

The food manufacturers have jumped on the probiotic bandwagon and there are supermarket shelves full of probiotics that contain more sugar than useful bacteria. These are often in the form of small yogurts or drinks, which are best avoided.

Vitamin D$_3$

Almost everybody that I test is either at the lower end, or deficient in vitamin D. It is critical for bone development, gut health, immunity and brain function. It can also boost your mood and help some dry skin conditions like eczema. Deficiency is often due to a poor diet and a lack of sun. Good food sources include oily fish, eggs and mushrooms.

However, sun exposure is the best source of vitamin D. The body finds it very hard to make vitamin D by itself and foods don't provide all our vitamin D needs. Due to the sun safety campaigns that warned us all about the dangers of skin cancer, many of us are now terrified of the sun and either avoid it altogether or cover ourselves in (toxic) sun cream, which can then result in a vitamin D deficiency. Of course it's sensible to protect yourself from the sun, especially if you are abroad in a hot country or outside in the midday sun for long periods. Babies, young children and

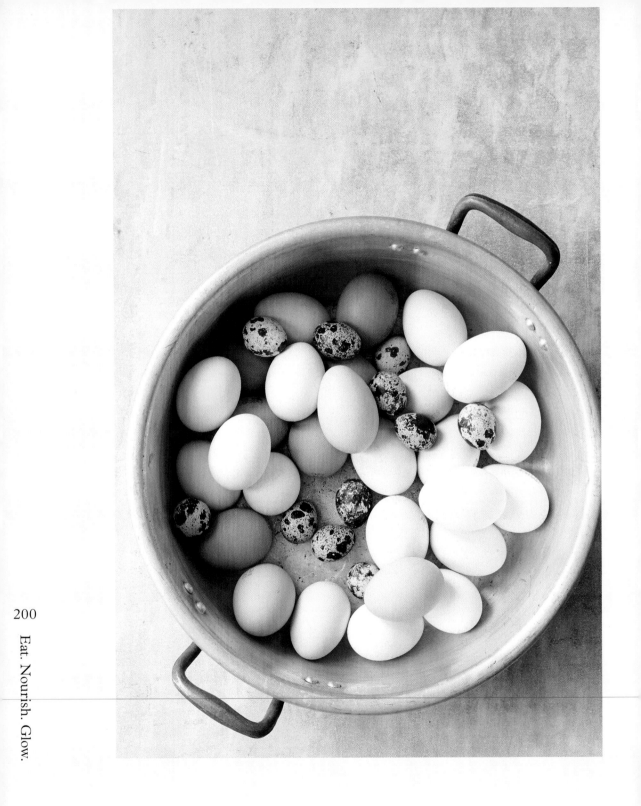

Eat. Nourish. Glow.

the elderly should be particularly careful not to burn. However, when it comes to adults a little bit of sensible sun exposure is a fantastic thing for your health. Fifteen or twenty minutes of sun a day helps your body make a huge amount of vitamin D. This is especially important from September through April when there isn't as much sun and daylight, so try and get out every day when it's bright. If the weather allows it, expose your arms, legs, chest and face to the sun so you make as much vitamin D as possible. The way that I work is always with the aim of optimal health, so I regularly take and suggest a vitamin D_3 supplement in liquid or capsule form for those who are deficient or have insufficient levels. However, it is essential to get your vitamin D levels checked to avoid toxicity.

Essential fatty acids

Most people, even those eating plenty of oily fish, nuts and seeds every week, don't get enough of these important fats to protect our health. The reason they are called essential fatty acids is because the body can't make them so it's essential we get them through diet and supplements. They protect our entire cellular health and are known to have anti-inflammatory, cancer-protecting and mood-boosting benefits as well as improving the quality and appearance of our skin, hair and nails. They also cushion our joints from wear and tear. There isn't a single function that essential fatty acids don't support. But again, quality is key. As the main source of essential fatty acids, also known as omega oils, is fish, you don't want to be swallowing mercury or PCBs (polychlorinated biphenyls) daily. You can also get some omega-3 from flaxseed oil if you prefer not to take a fish source, but it's not as beneficial as a fish oil supplement. So the better the quality, the less toxic they are. Always store them in the fridge to protect the oils.

201

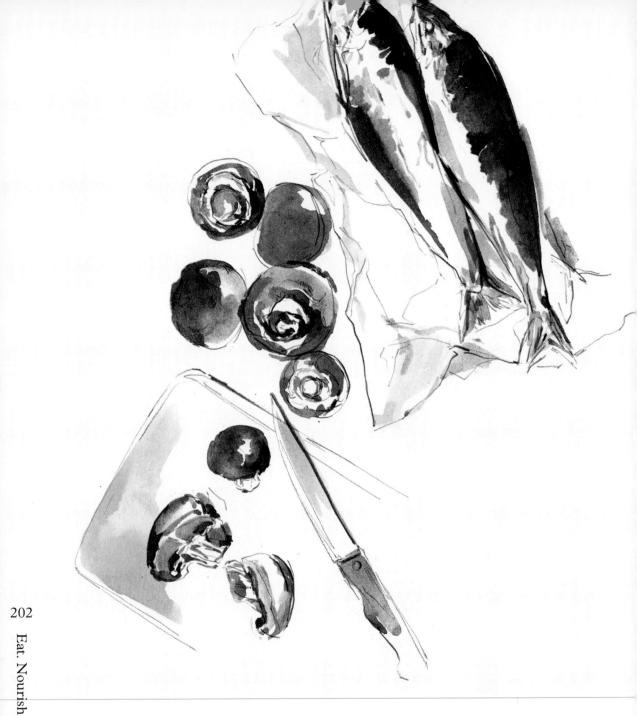

This chapter isn't a prescription as such, but a suggestion for those who wish to supplement their diets. In my experience supplements have proven to be so powerful in helping my clients—and myself, but they must be used carefully and wisely—don't take suggestions from anyone who isn't qualified and trained in their use.

CHAPTER 9
IN A NUTSHELL

If you decide to supplement your diet, do your research, seek advice from an expert and buy the best.

Keep moving—the importance of exercise for physical and mental health / Fitness snacking / Rethink movement and exercise / Make a plan and stick to it

Movement.

—No. 10

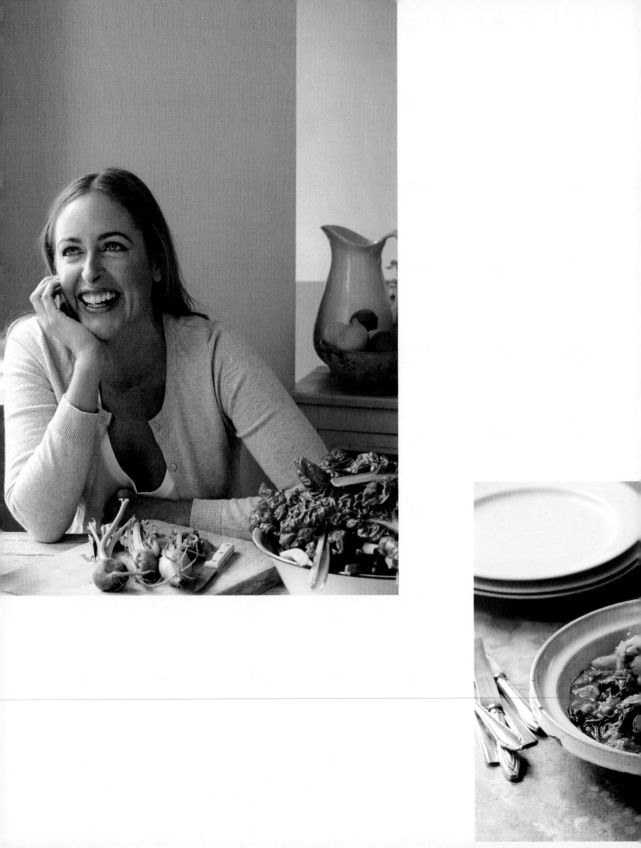

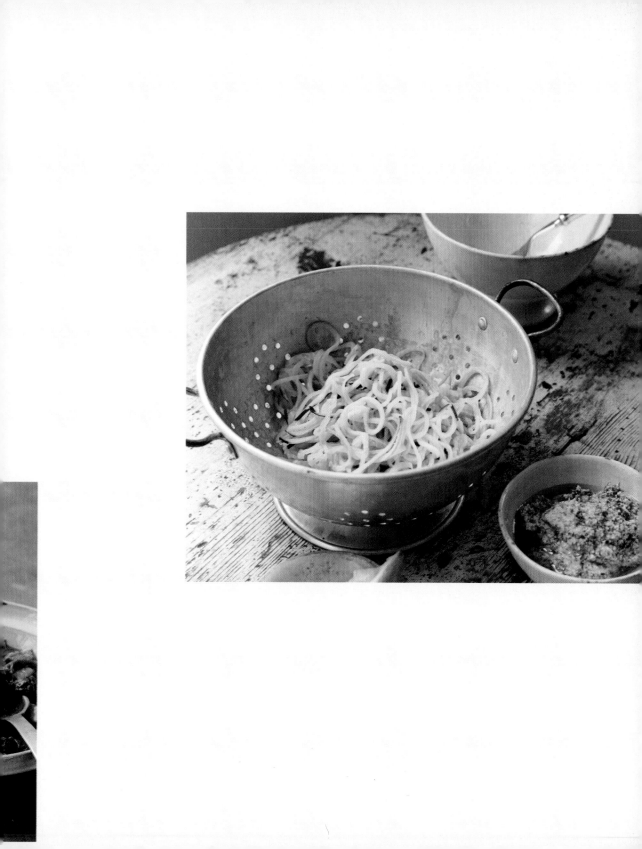

"If you have time for Facebook, you have time for exercise."

This may be the last chapter but it is by no means the least in terms of importance for our health. It's at the end because I firmly believe that you can't out-train a bad diet and so getting the diet sorted out first is key and then movement. To be truly healthy we have to move our bodies. It's that simple and there's absolutely no getting around it. We are created to move, not sit down—from the bus, to the chair, to the train, to the sofa—day in day out. I see in my practice that exercise, like food, has started to get problematic. There are some of us who avoid it and some of us who overdo it. Few find a healthy balance. In the same way that obsessive diets have created a web of confusing and complicated food fears in our heads, exercise and our relationship with it can also head that way—whether you are overdoing or underdoing it—both are equally bad for your health.

The truth? You don't have to spend a lot of money or time to move your body and be fit. It doesn't have to be complicated, intimidating, obsessive or stressful. It must be enjoyable.

On a functional medical course a few years ago, there was a lecture purely on exercise and the complexities of our relationship with it. One thing that really resonated with me was a fear of exercise. Intense exercise does not make me feel fantastic, awake and energetic—I don't get the endorphin high that people rave about. I hated PE at school and I can't stand being inside a gym. It makes me exhausted and for years I begrudgingly did it filled with hate. I developed quite a fear of it. I had some joint issues that meant the type of exercise I was doing was making things worse and more painful than actually beneficial. My whole attitude toward it was one of humiliation, discomfort and frustration. I know I'm not alone. I have many clients who find exercise a chore that makes them feel bad about themselves. Equally, there are many who overdo it in quite an obsessive way. After eight years of working with people and their health, trust me, I have heard all of the excuses and I know how to spot unhealthy relationships with food and exercise!

The lecturer at the conference said she had started to replace the word "exercise" with all its drab connotations with the phrase "gentle movement therapy." I love this and use it with my clients. When combined with good eating, physical activity is one of the more powerful ways to transform and optimize our health:

Its role in brain function is well established, particularly depression, Alzheimer's and Parkinson's disease.

Naturally it supports bone and joint health—think strong not skinny.

It is also well documented for its immune-boosting effects.

It supports healthy digestive functions.

It's a great way to reduce stress, improve self-esteem and sleep issues.

The NHS states that regular exercise—or movement therapy if you prefer to call it—can also lower your risk of diabetes, heart disease and cancer by up to a staggering 50 percent (visit www.health.gov/paguidelines or www.fitness.gov/resource-center/facts-and-statistics/). If exercise were a pill it would cost a fortune and we would all rush out to buy it, so what are you waiting for?

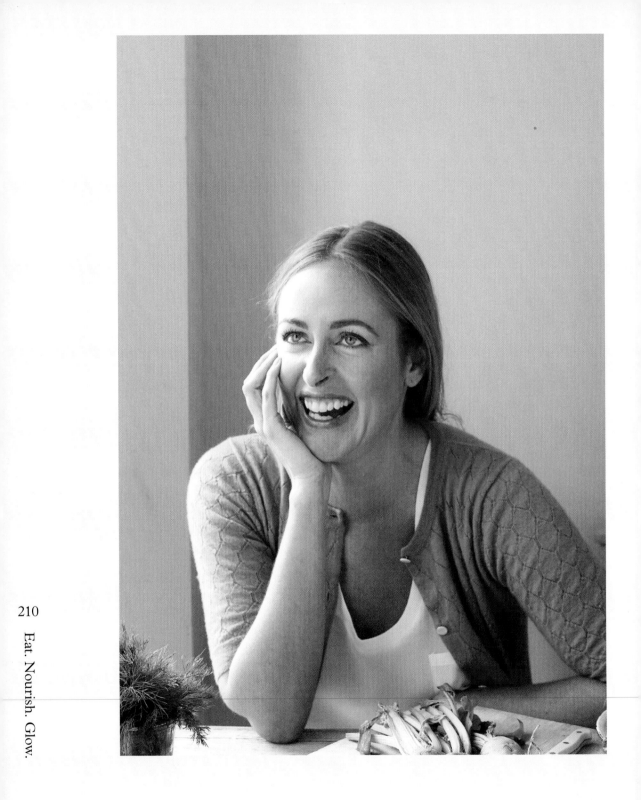

Eat. Nourish. Glow.

> "The six best doctors anywhere, and no one can deny it, are sunshine, water, rest, air, exercise and diet."

Wayne Fields

Fitness snacking

Research has emerged over the last few years telling us that we no longer need to slog it out in the gym for a whole hour at a time, as this way of exercising is, in fact, not so beneficial. "Fitness snacking" is where it's at! A study from Aberdeen University found that short bursts of intensive exercise scattered throughout the week burned more fat than longer but less frequent sessions. If your excuse has been lack of time for the hour-long gym classes or runs, then fitness snacking is your answer. Maybe we can just start off more simply than the fitness industry has led us to believe, for example, perhaps invest in a bike and ride it to go shopping or to work? Or go for a quick 10-minute jog when you get home? Or learn the basics of yoga and do some stretches before bed and when you wake up? Getting fit doesn't have to mean expensive personal trainers or gym memberships. I'm not saying that those of you who do enjoy an hour at a time at the gym must stop—please don't—the best kind of exercise is the one that you enjoy and if it's working for you then great, carry on, so long as you are challenging yourself out of your comfort zone when doing it.

One of the main reasons for lack of exercise, and another I personally relate to, is lack of results. Annoyingly we don't get the toned arms or six-pack after three or four sessions! So, in order to "flip" our thoughts and feelings about exercise, we must change the reason why we do it in the first place. I now do "movement therapy" just for me. It feels like decadent and indulgent "me" time, a space and an escape from my busy life. I do what I want to do and I enjoy it—by my own rules. I don't want to talk to anyone or share it with anyone, it's just time with me. It's more of a prescription that works with my mentality. One day I hope I will get the defined arms I long for or the toned bottom I used to have, but until then, I'm doing it for my brain, for my stress management and for my future. We simply need to change the way we think about movement. Its benefits are multiple and proven so take your pick!

> "Those who think they have no time for exercise will sooner or later have to find time for illness."

Edward Stanley

Rethink movement and exercise

If this book has convinced you to take pride and care in the foods you choose, then I hope you can extend this to exercise too—it's way beyond just making you feel and look amazing. If you have never been a fan of exercise, try to look at how you approach it, how you think about it, what you want to achieve out of it and how you can monitor your progress. In the same way I discussed about associating healthy food with happiness, do the same with exercise. If you start it with a mindset of dread and fear then it will be just that. Instead, think of exercise or movement as self-care, feel proud and make sure you enjoy what you do. If you hate running, don't run—find a local dance or yoga class instead. If the gym intimidates or bores you, don't go. Find a friend and exercise together instead—go running or play tennis. If you prefer being alone get a bike and start cycling. If you have a garden, get moving in it. If you work in an office, walk over to people to chat to them rather than sending them an email. Get out at lunchtime for a quick walk around the block. Leave your car behind and start to walk. Take the stairs—always. Get off the tube or bus a few stops early. I know these things in isolation are a little step but movement is essential and there are many ways to gradually build it into our lives.

Make sure when you start that you don't set the bar too high. Just like the juice cleanse or the extreme restriction diet—none of them are sustainable long term. If you start off working out too hard, causing exhaustion, injury and pain then you are more likely to give up! In our quest for the quickest, fastest results we throw ourselves into it and fall flat on our faces. It's exactly the same as the "I'll start the diet on Monday" mentality—hardly a way to create a long-term habit is it?

As a reminder—you can't out-train a bad diet! Exercise does not cancel out poor food choices or alcohol binges. While a reward has been shown to be beneficial when starting new exercise regimes, exercise is not an excuse to eat and drink all you want. You may tell yourself that but it's not. Sorry. Eating real food and physical activity are a beautiful combination—that's the aim.

Last, I also apply all the principles I have discussed in this book to exercise, for example, be consistent not perfect. If you are consistently moving your body every day then it's fine to have a lazy Sunday on the sofa. What you shouldn't have is a lazy week, every week, where you spend most of your time sitting at your desk or on the sofa. Be mindful and don't get stuck in a rut. Albert Einstein said insanity is doing the same thing over and over again and expecting different results. So if you have been going to the same aerobics class once a week for years then it's time to try something different. If you mainly focus on cardio then try some weights, yoga or Pilates instead. If you do Pilates all the time, try going for a run. We have to get out of our comfort zones with movement, so instead of giving up one thing (as in Chapter One), take up one thing and every day improve how you do that one thing, for example, a walk around the block or field. Time how long it takes you and each day knock off a minute and gradually expand the area you walk. Along with your kitchen detox, have a gym bag detox. Throw out your old sweaty beat-up trainers and treat yourselves to some bright new ones and strut around showing everyone how proud you are to be moving and taking care of yourself.

It's key to make a plan. Write a list of ways that you can realistically move your body day to day. Work out how to reward yourself for your efforts—make it a real reward for you. Studies show that after only 10 days your brain gets rewired to associate the exercise itself as a positive experience. Work out how you want to feel, then plan a goal—something you want to work toward. Work out how you plan to monitor your progress. Don't compete with anyone but yourself. If you fail to plan, you plan to fail!

CHAPTER 10 · IN A NUTSHELL

No magic potions, no fairy dust, no one to push you, no one to do it for you. Just one determined foot in front of the other. move your body!

Your toolkits.

So many of us feel daunted at the prospect of changing our diets. How will we find the time to think about what we are going to eat, let alone have the energy to prepare it? We feel scared of cooking unless we have ample time on our hands and step-by-step recipes to follow. It's all too easy to resort to the processed ready-made meals after a busy day at work, so I have put these toolkits together in an effort to illustrate the idea I live by, which is called food assembly. It's not rocket science, you don't need to be a gourmet chef and you don't need to spend a fortune. It's a question of thinking about the building blocks and types of fresh ingredients that amplify good health. Each toolkit shows you how to make a smoothie, salad or soup. Experiment with different vegetables and fruits, use a rainbow of colors, remember to include a protein source every time and work with a variety of herbs and spices to add flavor. Following these simple building blocks you will quickly gain confidence in whizzing up a quick smoothie for breakfast or a healthy salad/soup for lunch. Your old ways of eating will quickly be forgotten as your newfound energy from eating a fresh diet puts a spring in your step and a glow in your cheeks. Give it a try and see what you can create.

Smoothies

Choose:
a protein
+ 1 portion
   of fruit
+ some green
   vegetables
+ a liquid

Salads

Choose:
some leaves
+ 3 or 4 colored
  vegetables/fruits
+ some protein
+ a dressing

Eat. Nourish. Glow.

Soups

Choose:
<u>some basic flavors</u>
+ <u>a stock</u>
+ <u>some vegetables</u>
+ <u>a protein</u>
+ <u>some herbs</u>

Almond, apricot and rose "yogurt" /
Baked apples with vanilla coconut
cream / Beef curry / Buckwheat toast
with harissa "butter," sauerkraut and
poached egg / Cauliflower pizza with
roasted vegetables and pesto / Chicken
nuggets with mango and avocado salsa /
Creamy coffee milkshake / Crunchy
crab salad / Hazelnut chocolate salted
caramels / Lemon coconut mousse /
Lentil, beet and hazelnut salad with a
ginger dressing / Parsnip fritters /
Rainbow sandwich / Pear and prune
breakfast bowl with chia seeds and
apple / Raw chocolate marshmallows /
Super simple chicken and fries /
Steamed monkfish with a broccoli and
ginger mash / Smoked mackerel pâté

Recipes.

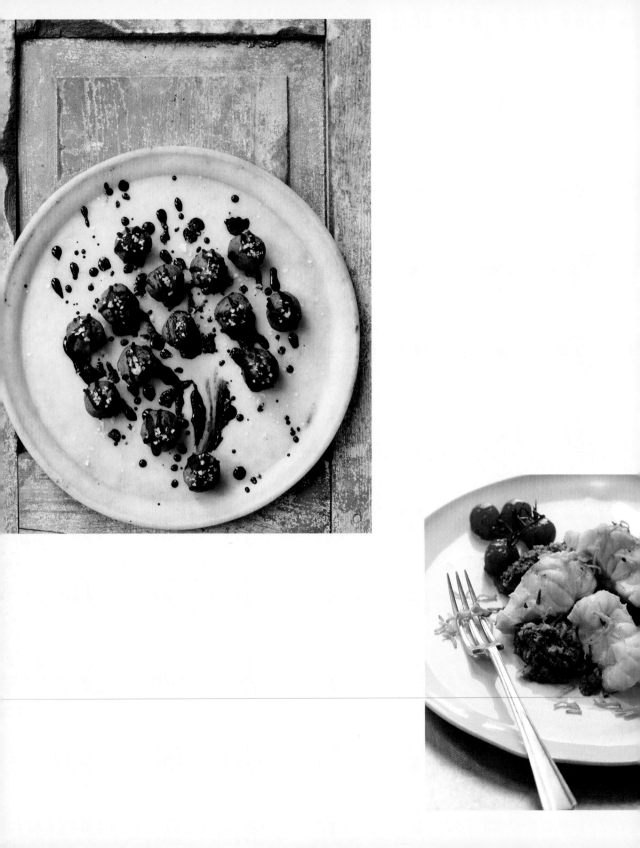

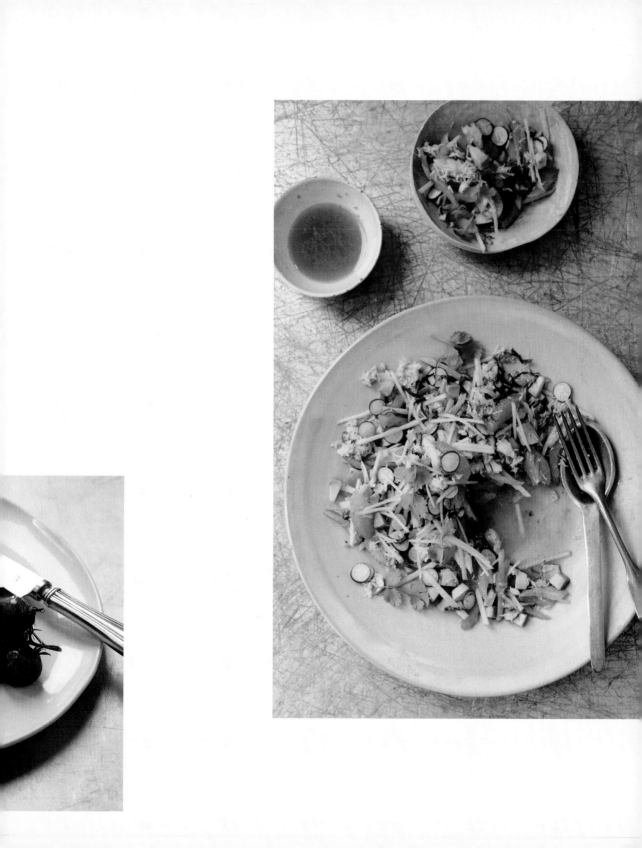

Almond, apricot and rose "yogurt"

Almonds and apricots used to be my favorite snack as they go so well together, so I thought why not blend them and see what happens? The result is a yummy, zingy, creamy combination that feels like a naughty dessert. I have also added a little rose water, which works perfectly as a delicious breakfast alternative to a sugary yogurt.

Prep time: 5 minutes
Soak time: 30 minutes or overnight
⅔ cup almonds
5 dried apricots
2 cardamom seeds
½ tsp rose water
1 tbsp unflavored coconut oil
1 cup coconut milk
2 fresh apricots, pitted and cut into quarters
Flaked almonds, for sprinkling

Soak the almonds in a bowl of cold water for 30 minutes, or overnight.
In another bowl, soak the apricots, cardamom and rose water for 30 minutes, or overnight.

When ready to serve, drain all the soaked ingredients, put into a blender, add the coconut oil and milk and blend until it is a creamy texture. Divide the mixture evenly between 2 jars or glasses, then top with the fresh apricots and a sprinkling of flaked almonds.

Put in the fridge and serve chilled.

—Serves 2

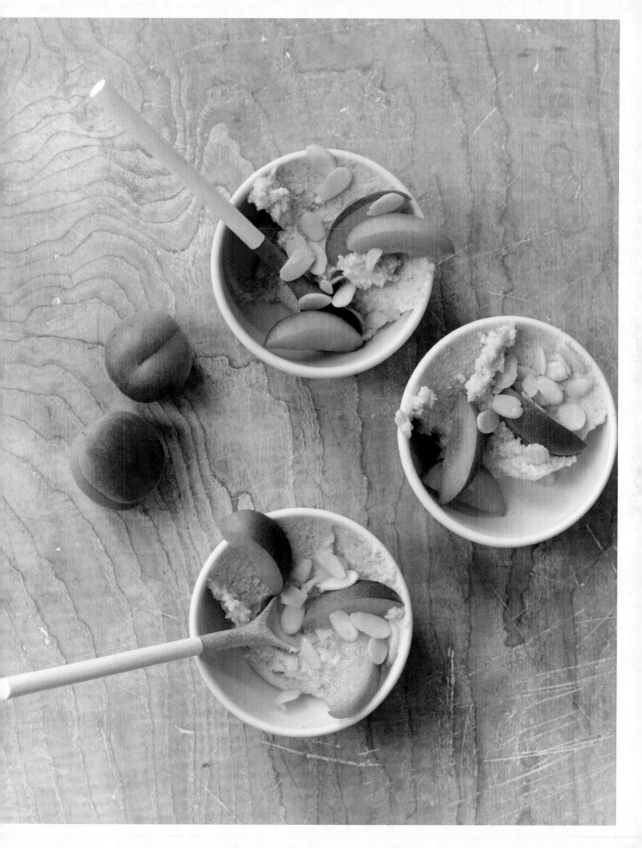

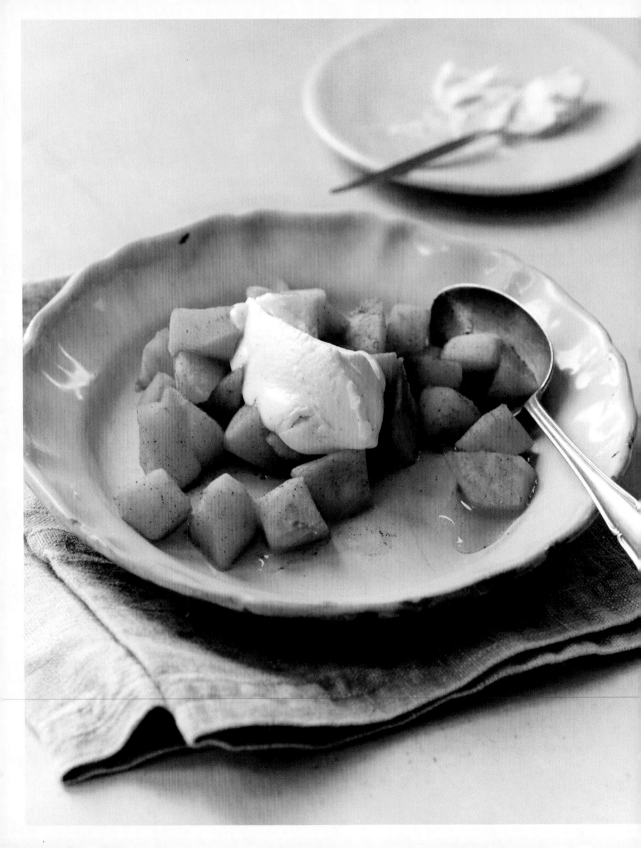

Baked apples with vanilla coconut cream

Apples are a brilliant source of prebiotics, which help good bacteria thrive in the gut, and this dish has great anti-inflammatory properties. Add a little vanilla coconut cream and you have a decadent treat for the most discerning!

Prep time: 15 minutes
Cook time: 15 minutes

4 organic apples, peeled and chopped into bite-sized cubes
1 tsp ground cinnamon
1 tsp vanilla extract or powder (available online)
2 x 13.5-oz cans coconut milk, cooled in the fridge for 3 hours minimum

Preheat the oven to 300°F.

Place the apples in a heavy-based, ovenproof dish and sprinkle with the cinnamon and a little water. Bake in the oven for 15 minutes until soft.

Meanwhile, remove the top creamy part of the coconut milk from the cans and place in a bowl. Add the vanilla and whisk until smooth and creamy.

Keep in the fridge until ready to serve.

To serve, spoon the cooked apple into four ramekins and put a dollop of cream on top.

Note

You can add probiotic powders to this dessert to enhance its gut healing properties, if you wish.

—Serves 2

Beef curry

I make this curry in my slow cooker but it works just as well in a casserole. I love to have melt in the mouth, tender meat and so the slow cooker is ideal for this. It's just so easy but feels like a really delicious hearty meal—great for a Friday night with friends. Everyone always thinks that they need to have rice or bread with a curry but I add lots of vegetables, so it's actually more than enough on its own. I sometimes serve this curry with cauliflower rice, which works very well.

Prep time: 10–15 minutes
Cook time: 5–8 hours 20 minutes (3 hours if using a conventional oven preheated to 300°F)

1 lb organic stewing steak, cut into cubes
2 x 13.5 oz cans organic coconut milk
1 large onion, peeled and diced
2 garlic cloves, keep whole (to remove at the end)
1-inch cube of fresh ginger, peeled and cut into thin slices
2 small red chilies, finely sliced (I keep the seeds in as I like the heat but remove for a milder version)
3 star anise
2 tbsp ground cumin
2 tbsp ground coriander
1 cup fresh beef or chicken stock or water
2 sweet potatoes, peeled and cut into bite-sized chunks
10 cherry tomatoes
⅕ cup fresh spinach
1 tbsp fish sauce
Sea salt and freshly ground black pepper
Fresh cilantro, to serve

Put all of the ingredients except the sweet potatoes, tomatoes, spinach and fish sauce into the slow cooker. Stir and add a generous pinch of salt and pepper.

Set the slow cooker to high, cover with the lid and leave to cook for 5 hours. Alternatively, set the slow cooker to low and leave to cook overnight.

Before serving, add the sweet potatoes, tomatoes and fish sauce and cook for a further 20 minutes, then stir in the spinach.

Sprinkle the cilantro over the top and serve.

—Serves 2

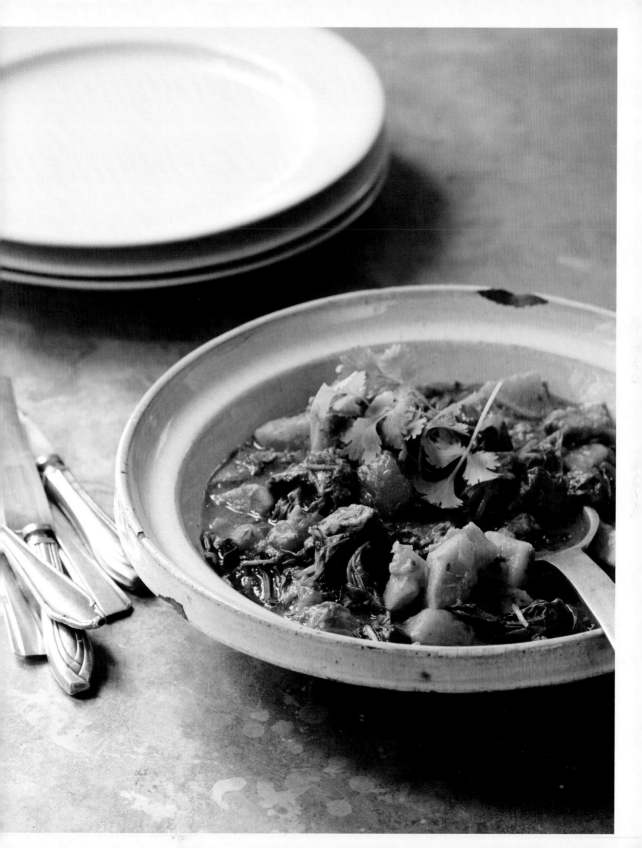

Buckwheat toast with harissa "butter," sauerkraut and poached egg

Eggs and chilies are a winning combination for me. Sauerkraut is such a fantastic food that helps to encourage healthy bacteria to thrive in our digestive system and it just works well with this combination. I'm always trying to get vegetables into all three meals so this is a great way. This recipe is equally lovely with raw fennel and lamb's lettuce.

Prep time: 2 minutes
Cook time: 3–5 minutes

1 tsp white wine vinegar (optional)
1 organic egg
1 slice of gluten-free bread of choice
1 tsp unflavored coconut butter or ghee
½ tsp homemade harissa (see page 76) or a good-quality bought
   one will also work)
2 tbsp sauerkraut (either homemade or a good-quality, unpasturized one)

Poach your egg. Half-fill a wide saucepan with cold water, add the vinegar (if using) and bring to the boil. Crack the egg into a ramekin and carefully slide it into the water where you can see bubbles. Poach for about 2–3 minutes, or until the white is set, then remove with a slotted spoon, pat dry on kitchen paper and trim the ragged edges with a sharp knife.

Meanwhile, toast the bread. If using buckwheat bread, it may need to be toasted a couple of times until it is crisp.

In a small bowl, mix the coconut butter or ghee with the harissa spice mix (see page 76), then spread the butter on the toast and layer the sauerkraut over it. Put the egg on top.

—Serves 1

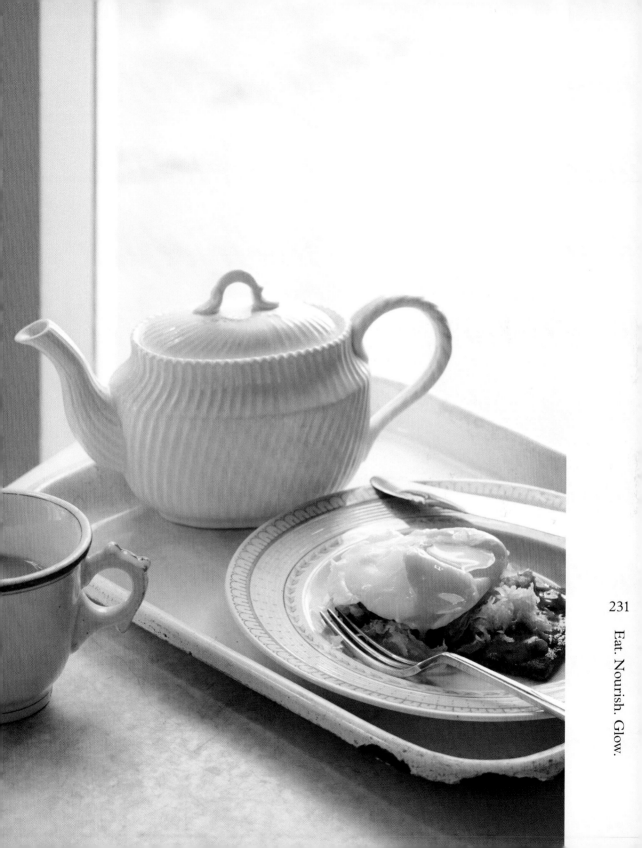

231

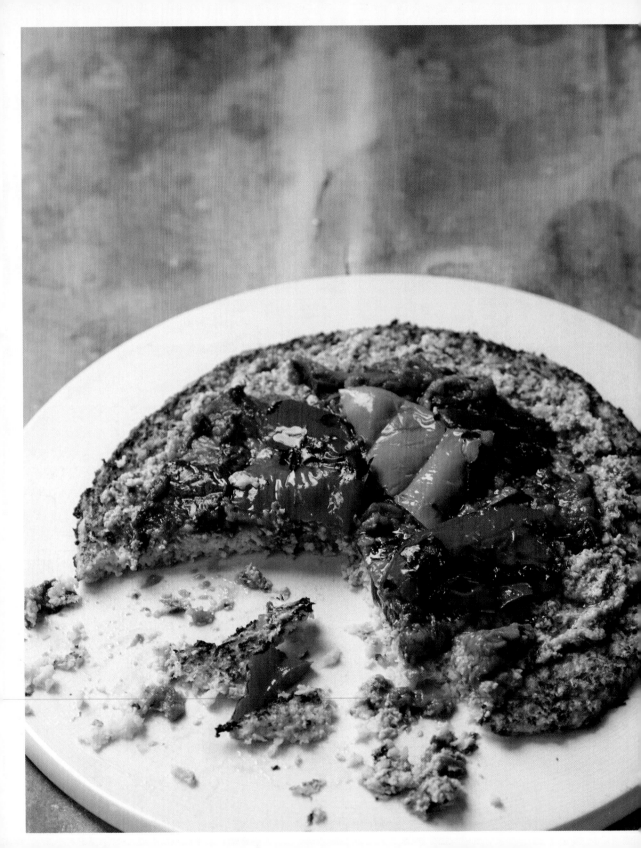

Cauliflower pizza with roasted vegetables and pesto

The words "nutritious" and "pizza" can finally be used together with this wonderful combination. No gluten or wheat in sight when you serve up this cauliflower specialty . . . choose your toppings and enjoy!

Prep time: 10 minutes
Cook time: 15 minutes

coconut oil, for greasing
1 lb cauliflower, washed, dried and blitzed in a blender into small "rice"
1 egg
a pinch of sea salt and freshly ground black pepper
1 tbsp gluten-free flour (I use brown rice flour)
1 tsp nutritional yeast flakes
2 tsp Italian seasoning

To serve:
Homemade herby pesto (see page 80)
Roasted eggplant and peppers

Preheat the oven to 325°F. Grease the baking sheet with coconut oil, then line it with parchment paper and grease this too.

Steam the cauliflower rice for 3–4 minutes. Don't let it get mushy, then put it in a tea towel and squeeze out all of the excess water.

Put the cauliflower rice into a large bowl, add the egg, seasoning, flour and yeast flakes and mix well.

Spoon the mixture—it should still be a little wet—over the lined baking sheet and spread it out evenly over the paper. Make sure there are no holes in the mixture.

Bake in the oven for 40 minutes, or until golden and crisp. Remove from the baking sheet and leave to air for a few minutes.

To serve, spread over a little herby pesto and arrange some roasted eggplant and peppers over the top.

—Serves 2–3

Chicken nuggets with mango and avocado salsa

Here's a recipe for the whole family, a healthy version of chicken nuggets. Throw in a good measure of childhood nostalgia and enjoy.

Prep time: 10 minutes
Chill time: 30 minutes
Cook time: 15 minutes

2 skinless chicken breasts, cut into cubes
1 cup coconut milk
½ cup coconut flour
½ tsp ground cumin
½ tsp tumeric powder
½ tsp ground coriander
⅓ cup desiccated coconut
A pinch of salt
1 tbsp coconut oil, melted
4 large lettuce leaves from an iceberg or cos lettuce, to serve

Salsa:

1 avocado, peeled, stoned and cut into small cubes
1 mango, peeled, stoned and cut into small cubes
1 tbsp fresh cilantro, torn
1 red onion, peeled and finely diced
1 red chili, finely diced
2 tbsp coconut aminos

Put the chicken cubes in a bowl with the coconut milk and refrigerate for 30 minutes.

Meanwhile, make the mango salsa. Mix the avocado, mango, cilantro, onion and chili together in a bowl and pour over the coconut aminos. Refrigerate until needed.

Preheat the oven to 350°F.

Put the flour and spices in a bowl and put the desiccated coconut on a plate.

Take a chicken cube, roll it in the spiced flour, then roll it in the desiccated coconut until it is well coated, then put it on a baking tray. Repeat with the remaining chicken cubes.

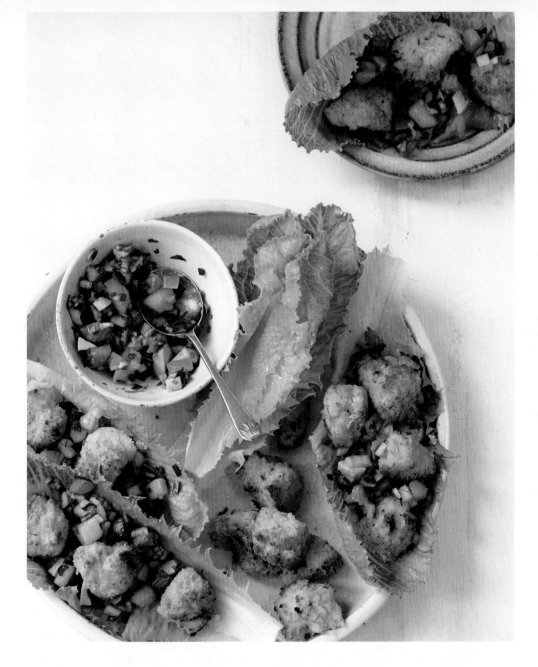

Pour the melted coconut oil over the chicken and bake in the oven for
15 minutes, or until the chicken is cooked through, golden brown and crispy.

To serve, put a spoonful of the mango salsa into each lettuce leaf, add a
few chicken nuggets, fold in the sides of the lettuce to enclose it and eat like
a sandwich.

—Serves 2–3

Creamy coffee milkshake

We all know how much we like our coffee in the morning, well here's a healthy version that will wake-up your taste buds as well as delivering a gelatin protein boost. You will know you are onto a good thing.

Prep time: 5 minutes
Freeze time: 30 minutes

Protein cubes:
1 tbsp grass-fed gelatin powder (can be bought online)
½ cup organic canned coconut milk
1 cup hot espresso
½ tsp coconut crystals (optional)
A small pinch of sea salt

Milkshake:
1 cup espresso
1 cup coconut milk
1 tbsp coconut butter
A pinch of vanilla powder
4 protein cubes
4 ice cubes

For the protein cubes, sprinkle the gelatin over the cold coconut milk and stir until the gelatin has dissolved and a paste has formed. Leave to rest for a few minutes, then pour the hot espresso on top and stir.

Add the coconut crystals (if using) and the salt, then pour the mixture into ice-cube trays. Freeze for 30 minutes to cool.

This makes more than enough protein cubes so you have extra for other days.

To make the milkshake, put all the ingredients into the blender and blend until combined. Serve.

—Serves 1–2

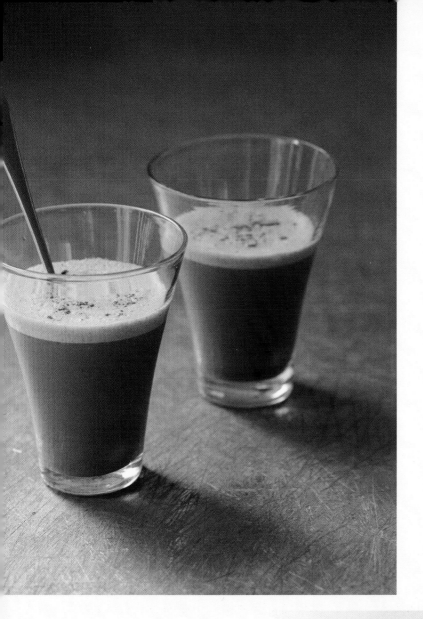

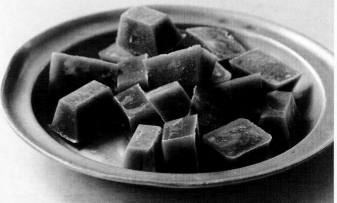

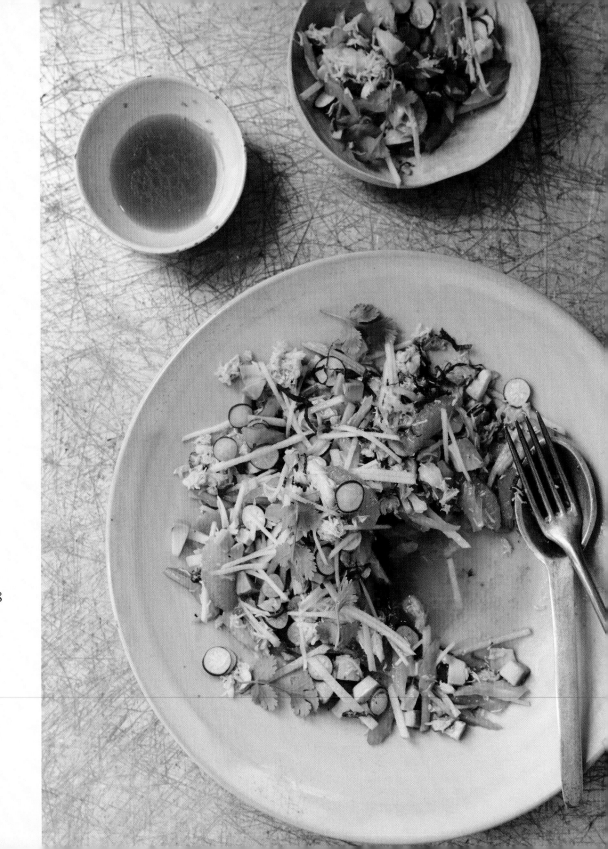

Eat. Nourish. Glow.

Crunchy crab salad

I love getting some color into my salads. In this recipe it's by adding some pink grapefruit and radishes. Combining fresh flavors with a good source of protein scores this salad top marks for energy and vitality.

Prep time: 10 minutes

½ lb fresh crabmeat

1 avocado, peeled, pitted and cut into small cubes

2 celery sticks, cut into small pieces

1 pink grapefruit, peeled and cut into segments, retain the juice

1 bunch of radishes, topped and tailed then cut into small sticks with
   a mandoline

1 Granny Smith apple, cored and cut into sticks with a mandoline

1 tsp fresh ginger root, peeled and cut into thin sticks (you can also
   juice and add to the dressing if you prefer)

A handful of fresh cilantro leaves

Half that amount of fresh mint leaves, cut into fine strips

For the dressing:

2 tbsp pink grapefruit juice

1 tbsp lemon juice

1 tsp salt

1 tsp fresh ginger juice

2 tbsp extra virgin olive oil

1 tsp coriander seeds, slightly toasted and crushed into a powder
   (ground coriander is fine if you don't have time)

Freshly cracked black pepper

To make the dressing, put the ginger and citrus juices into a bowl, add the salt and stir until dissolved. Add the ground coriander and pepper, then while whisking, slowly pour in the olive oil until combined.

Mix all the salad ingredients together in a large bowl, pour over the dressing and serve.

—Serves 2

Hazelnut chocolate salted caramels

Seriously decadent and truly delectable, these salted caramels are hard to resist. Make them to share with friends or when you know you won't be tempted to eat the lot!

Prep time: 15–20 minutes
Soak time: 20 minutes
Freeze time: 3 hours

14 small medjool dates, pitted
⅓ cup coconut milk
⅓ cup melted coconut oil
¼ tsp Maldon sea salt, plus sea salt flakes for sprinkling
½ tsp vanilla powder
12 raw hazelnuts
Coconut flour, for dusting

Chocolate coating:
5 tsp cocoa powder
5 tsp coconut oil
2 tbsp coconut crystals

Soak the dates in a bowl of hot water for 20 minutes, then drain and put them into a blender with the coconut milk, coconut oil, salt and vanilla powder. Blend into a smooth paste, then transfer to a freezerproof container and freeze for 1 hour.

Line a baking tray with greaseproof paper. Roll a hazelnut in the caramel mixture until it's coated—it's messy and the balls won't be a perfect shape but this doesn't matter, just keep using teaspoons to handle the caramel. Dust with a little coconut flour so the balls don't stick together and put onto the lined baking tray. Repeat until all the mixture is used up, then put the tray into the freezer and freeze for 3 hours.

While the nuts are freezing, make the chocolate coating. Put all the ingredients for the coating in a pan and set over a low heat, stirring until melted. Remove from the heat and leave the mixture to cool a little until it is thick enough to drizzle over the caramel balls.

Pour the coating over the caramel balls, sprinkle a little salt over each, then pop back into the freezer for 30 minutes.

—Makes 12 caramels

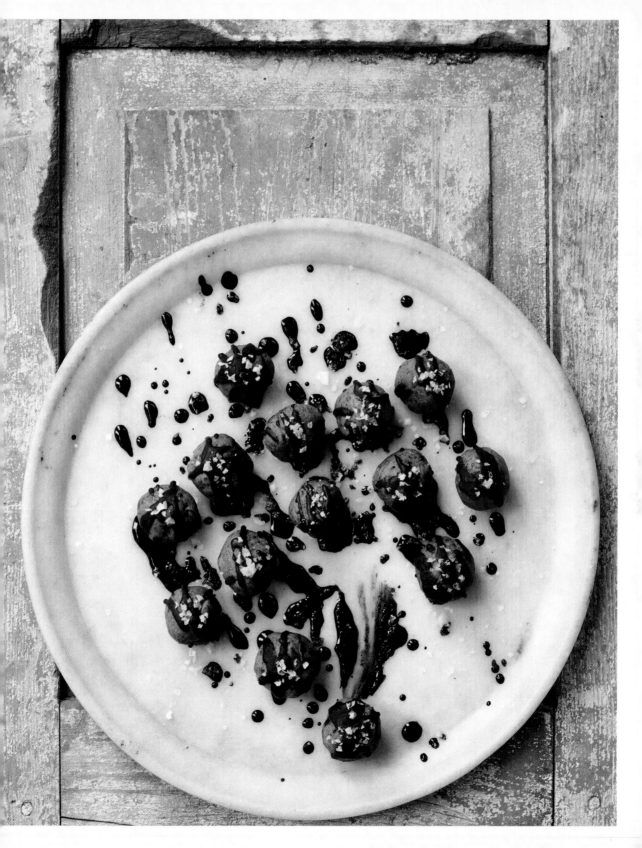

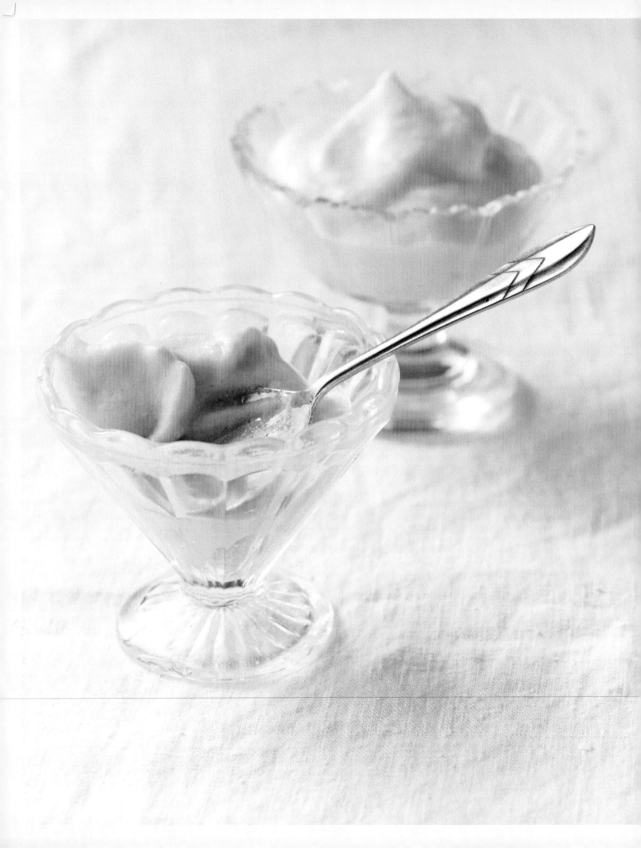

Lemon coconut mousse

If you like something a little sweet but appreciate that the processed fat-free yogurts in the supermarket do you no good at all, then try this alternative dessert. Light, fruity and all natural—it's a mousse to soothe the senses. Go on—indulge yourself.

Prep time: 15 minutes
Chill time: 4 ½ hours

13.5-oz can of coconut milk
3 medium eggs, separated
⅓ cup local organic honey (or less)
Juice and zest of 2 unwaxed organic lemons
A pinch of salt

Chill the coconut can in the fridge for at least 2 hours, so that the coconut cream floats to the top. You only need to use the cream, so keep the rest of the milk to flavor a soup or a smoothie.

Place the egg yolks, honey, lemon zest and lemon juice in a heatproof bowl set over a pan of simmering water and whisk constantly for about 10 minutes until the mixture thickens. Remove from the heat and chill in the fridge for about 30 minutes.

Meanwhile, scoop out the chilled coconut cream from the top of the can into a bowl and beat with a whisk or spoon until stiff.

In separate clean bowl, beat the egg whites and sea salt until stiff.

Fold the lemon mixture into the coconut cream, then gently fold in the egg whites.

Chill in the fridge for at least 2 hours, then spoon into pretty glasses or bowls to serve.

—Serves 3–4

Lentil, beet and hazelnut salad with a ginger dressing

Nourish your body with this welcoming salad complete with a warming ginger dressing. Lentils provide a fabulous source of protein and the beet adds that splash of color I love so much.

Prep time: 10 minutes
Cook time: 10 minutes

1 cup Puy lentils, rinsed
2¾ cup filtered water
Sea salt
3 cooked beets, cut into small cubes
2 spring onions, finely sliced
2 tbsp hazelnuts, roughly chopped
A handful of fresh mint, roughly chopped
A handful of fresh parsley, roughly chopped

Ginger dressing:
¾-inch cube of fresh ginger, peeled and roughly chopped
6 tbsp olive oil
1 tsp Dijon mustard
1 tbsp apple cider vinegar
Pinch of sea salt and freshly ground black pepper

For the lentils, put them in a saucepan, cover with water, bring to a boil then reduce the heat and simmer for about 15–20 minutes, or until all the liquid has evaporated and the lentils are not mushy and still with a bite.

As soon as the lentils are cooked transfer them to a large bowl and leave to cool.

Once the lentils are cool, add the beets, spring onions, hazelnuts and herbs and stir until everything is combined.

For the dressing, put the ginger, mustard, oil and vinegar in a bowl and, using a hand-held blender, blend until combined.

Drizzle the dressing over the salad and serve.

—Serves 2–3

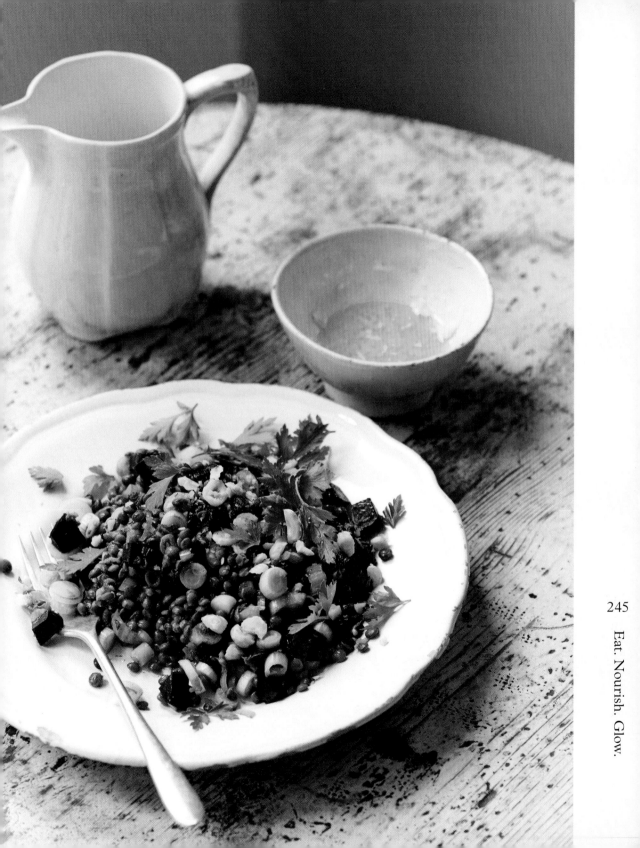

Eat. Nourish. Glow.

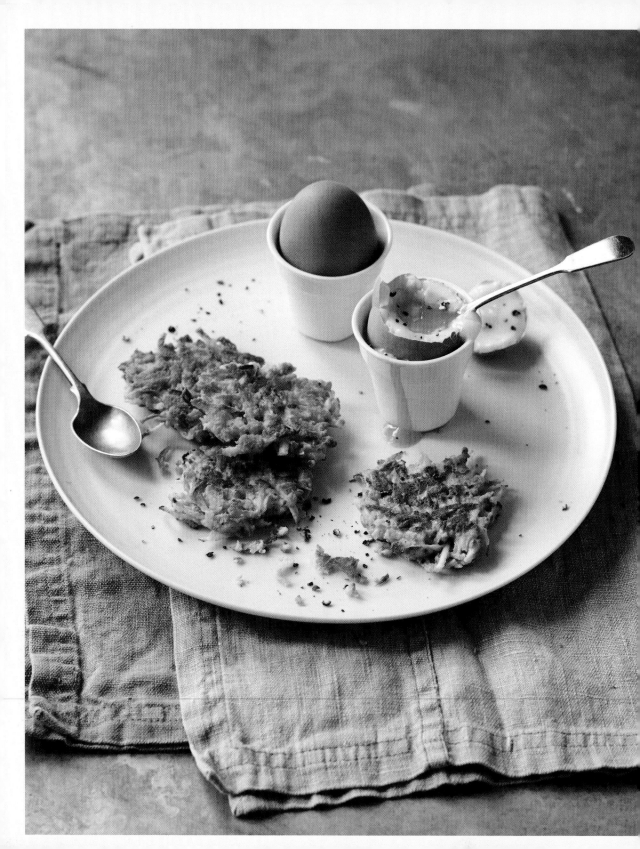

Parsnip fritters

A healthy version of the hash brown—but just as satisfying. These work just as well with zucchini or sweet potato and are lovely at any meal but I particularly love them with an egg for breakfast. I often add some spinach or avocado too.

Prep time: 15 minutes
Cook time: 15 minutes

1 parsnip, peeled and grated into sticks using a mandoline or grater
2 tbsp coconut flour
1 egg, beaten
1 tsp ground cumin
A pinch of sea salt and freshly ground black pepper
1 tbsp coconut oil, melted

For the fritters: mix all the ingredients together in a bowl until combined, then using your hands or a spoon, divide the mixture into 6 portions. Mold each portion together roughly.

Heat the coconut oil and fry the fritters for about 2 minutes on each side until crisp and golden brown. If you are making larger batches, you can also bake in the oven preheated to 325°F on a baking tray, covered in greaseproof paper. Serve.

—Makes 6 fritters

Rainbow sandwich

Let's face it, a sandwich is still the standard default at lunchtime so I thought I would create the healthiest one possible! This is not only the prettiest of sandwiches but it's bursting with flavor as well as nutrients. It's one of my favorite recipes. For those of you that don't want to eat the buckwheat bread, you can wrap the filling in a large salad or spring green leaf instead.

Prep time: 10 minutes

4 slices of buckwheat bread, lightly toasted (you can use a bread of choice or lettuce leaves)
1 tbsp pesto
1 tbsp artichoke paste
1 carrot, peeled and grated then mixed with a little lemon juice
2 cooked beets, peeled and very thinly sliced with a mandoline
4 radishes, thinly sliced with a mandoline (or grated)
1 yellow pepper, cut in half, then each half cut into 3 and grilled
½ red onion, peeled and thinly sliced with a mandoline
1 tomato, sliced into thin rounds
A small handful of watercress
6 fresh basil leaves
Fresh parsley, to taste
Sea salt and freshly ground black pepper

Spread one slice of toasted bread with the artichoke paste and the other with the pesto.

Layer the carrot on one slice, followed by the beets, the radishes, yellow pepper, red onion, tomato, then the watercress on top and finish with the herbs. Season with the salt and pepper. Put the other slice of bread on top and push down. Cut in half and serve. It's a bit messy but just get messy and enjoy it!

—Serves 2

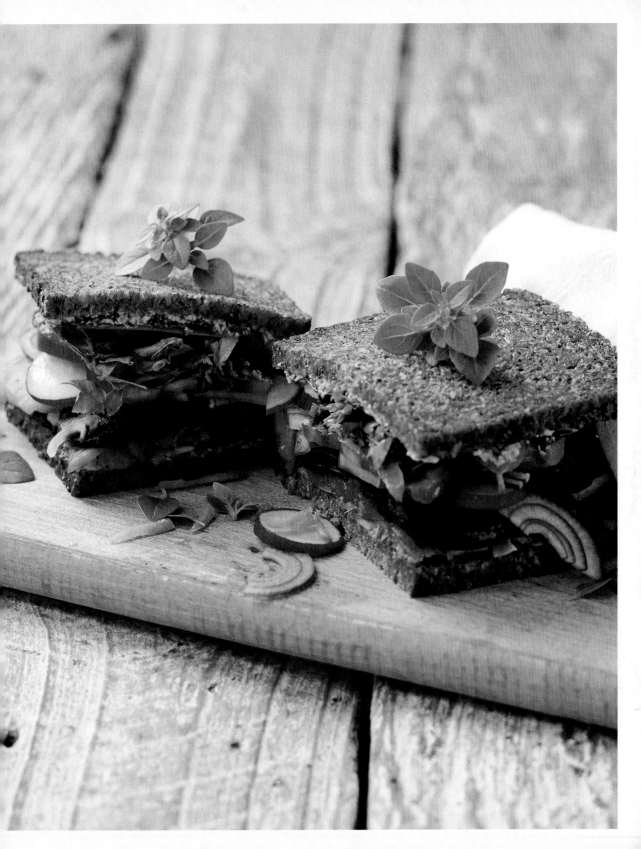

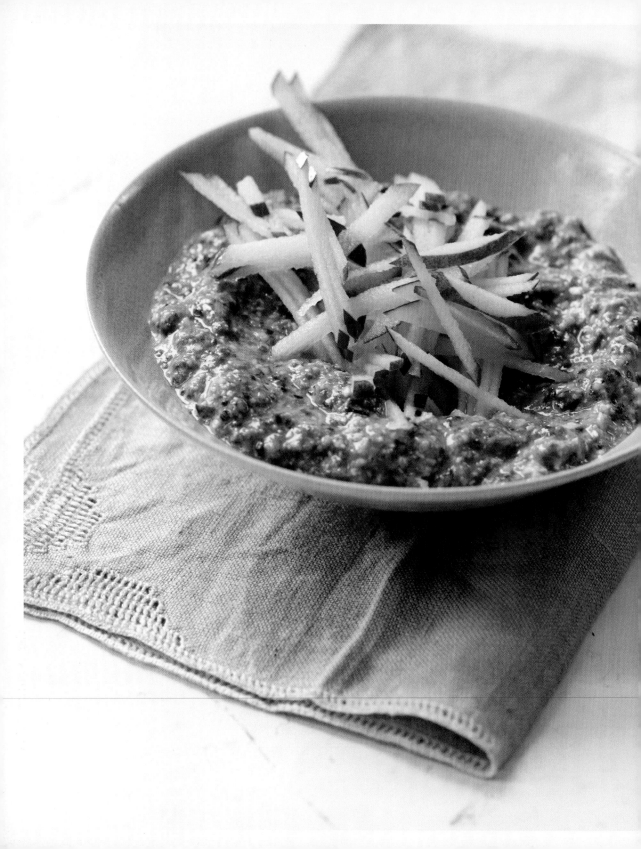

Pear and prune breakfast bowl with chia seeds and apple

What a lovely way to start the day. Chia seeds provide a good source of protein to keep you going until lunchtime so give your early morning metabolism a boost with this fruity, healthy alternative and lavish these mid-morning energy dips.

Prep time: 10 minutes
Soak time: 8 hours

2 ripe pears
6 dried prunes
6 tbsp fresh walnuts
Salt
1 tsp chia seeds
A tiny pinch of ground cinnamon
1 apple, cored and grated into matchsticks with a mandoline

Put the prunes and 1 cup filtered water in a bowl. In another bowl, put the walnuts and cover with salted filtered water and leave both to soak overnight. Drain.

The next day, drain the prunes reserving the liquid. Soak the chia seeds in the prune liquid for 20 minutes.

Put the pears, soaked prunes, walnuts, chia seeds and cinnamon into a blender and blend until smooth, adding some of the soaking prune water if necessary.

Pour the mixture into a small glass, jar or bowl, then add the apple matchsticks and serve.

—Serves 2

Raw chocolate marshmallows

These marshmallows are a bit of a revelation. Light, fluffy and gourmet you can almost be forgiven for thinking they must be a forbidden food but with these gems you get a gelatin protein boost that's great for your gut combined with a chocolate hit to heighten the feel-good factor. Don't forget they are a treat!

Prep time: 15 minutes
Set time: 2 hours

3 tbsp grass-fed gelatin powder
1 cup filtered water
½ cup coconut nectar
1 tsp vanilla extract
¼ tsp sea salt
Raw cacao powder, to serve

You will need a 20 x 20cm baking sheet

Line the baking sheet with parchment paper lengthways and then using another piece, line widthways, ensuring there is enough parchment paper overhanging the sides to cover the marshmallows.

Put the gelatin and ½ cup water in a freestanding mixer and mix until the gelatin is soft.

Meanwhile, pour the remaining ½ cup water into a saucepan along with the coconut nectar, vanilla and salt and bring the mixture to a boil. Boil the mixture for about 7–8 minutes, then immediately remove from the heat.

Turn your mixer to low (or you can use a hand-held whisk if it is too powerful) and slowly pour the coconut nectar mixture into the bowl combining it with the softened gelatin.

Turn the mixer to high and continue beating for about 10 minutes, or until the mixture becomes thick like marshmallow creme. Turn off the mixer and transfer the marshmallow creme to the prepared sheet. Smooth the top, then press it down with parchment paper. Leave until the marshmallow is completely set.

Cut the marshmallow to your desired size (I make small cubes) and dust with raw cacao powder to serve.

—Makes 16 marshmallows

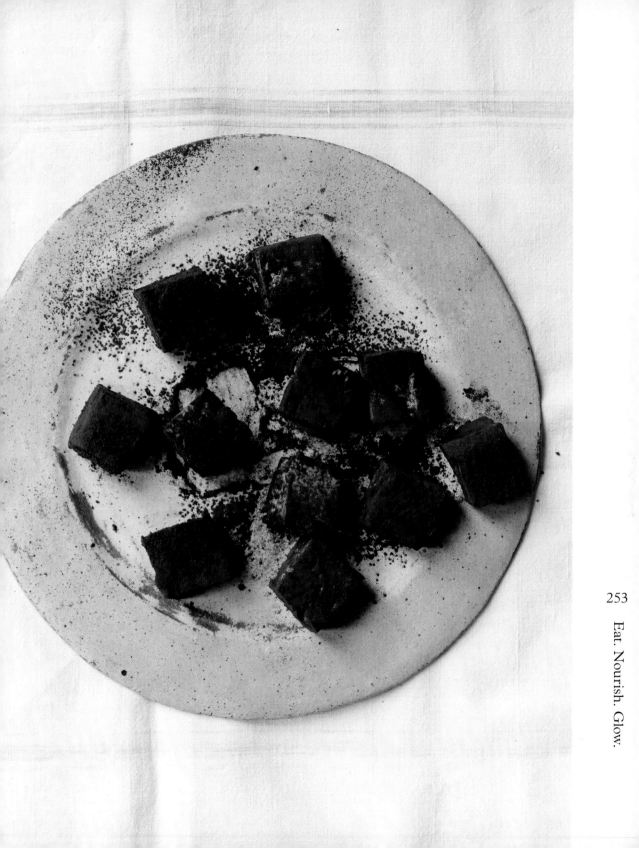

Eat. Nourish. Glow.

Super simple chicken and fries

I completely forgot about this dish that I used to make so often in my early days. In this process of creating recipes for the book, it is easy to get lost in trying to be really creative and original, but ultimately, my clients want simple and healthy recipes. I suddenly remembered this dish that I created when I was single and missing the roast chicken Sunday lunch, although I did make it many week nights. It's quick, easy, adaptable and to me, the epitome of comfort food. I hope you will enjoy making it for yourself, for a date night, for your kids or a Sunday special for friends and family—it's a completely no-fail recipe that certainly isn't my own invention but is absolutely a staple in my home for years to come.

Prep time: 10 minutes
Cook time: 20 minutes
1 chicken breast, cut into 6 thin strips
1–2 red chilies, finely chopped (seed and use 1 chili if you don't like heat)
1 large garlic clove, minced
Juice and zest of 1 lemon
2 tbsp unflavored coconut oil, plus extra olive or coconut oil for the chicken (optional)
1 sweet potato, peeled and shredded into thin sticks with a mandoline
2 tsp paprika
Sea salt or Himalyan salt and freshly ground black pepper

Put the chicken strips, chilies, garlic, lemon juice and zest in a large bowl and mix well. Cover and leave to marinate in the fridge for as long as possible (I often don't have time and just cook it immediately, but it is better if marinated for at least 30 minutes). Add a little olive or coconut oil if leaving overnight or longer than 3 hours.

Heat 1 tablespoon coconut oil in a frying pan over a medium heat. Add the potato sticks and fry, turning and moving continually—they are so fine that they can quickly and easily burn so keep an eye on them. Once browned on all sides and crisp, put them on a plate and cover with kitchen paper.

Using the same pan, heat a little more coconut oil, then add the chicken strips and fry on each side until golden brown and cooked. Turn off the heat, add about 2 tablespoons water and cover with a lid. This allows the chicken to cool slowly without getting too dry.

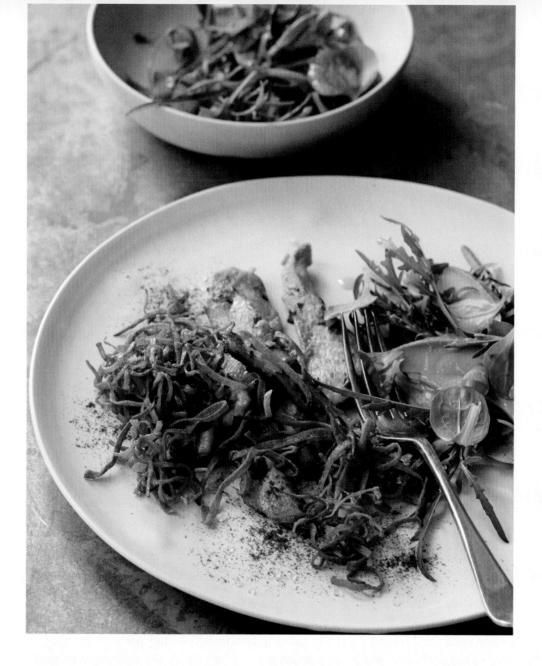

   Season with the paprika, salt and perpper and serve with a simple green salad such as arugula, lamb's lettuce and avocado with a mustard, olive oil and lemon dressing.

   To me, this is truly comfort food.

—Serves 2

Steamed monkfish with a broccoli and ginger mash

I used to love mashed potatoes, but this mashed broccoli is a perfect substitute—a healthy take on fish pie!

Prep time: 10 minutes
Cook time: 15 minutes

2 heads broccoli, broken into florets
1 tsp salt
2-inch piece of fresh ginger, peeled and cut into very fine matchsticks
2–3 tbsp coconut oil (flavorless or not)
A handful of fresh basil
1 red chili, seeded and roughly chopped
1 tbsp broccoli cooking water (see method)
1 tbsp fish sauce
1 lb monkfish
Grilled cherry tomatoes, to serve

Blanch the broccoli in a pan of salted boiling water for 3 minutes, then drain, reserving a tablespoon of the cooking water, and cool immediately under cold running water.

Gently fry the ginger matchsticks in the coconut oil over low heat for 2 minutes. Turn off the heat and let the ginger infuse a little longer.

Blend the broccoli with the ginger flavored coconut oil and a little of the ginger (reserve some ginger for the garnish), the basil, chili, the reserved cooking water and the fish sauce.

Salt the monkfish and steam for 8–10 minutes, or until cooked.

Reheat the broccoli mash until hot, then spoon it onto two plates. Put the monkfish on top and sprinkle with the reserved crispy ginger sticks. Serve immediately with the grilled cherry tomatoes on the side.

—Serves 2

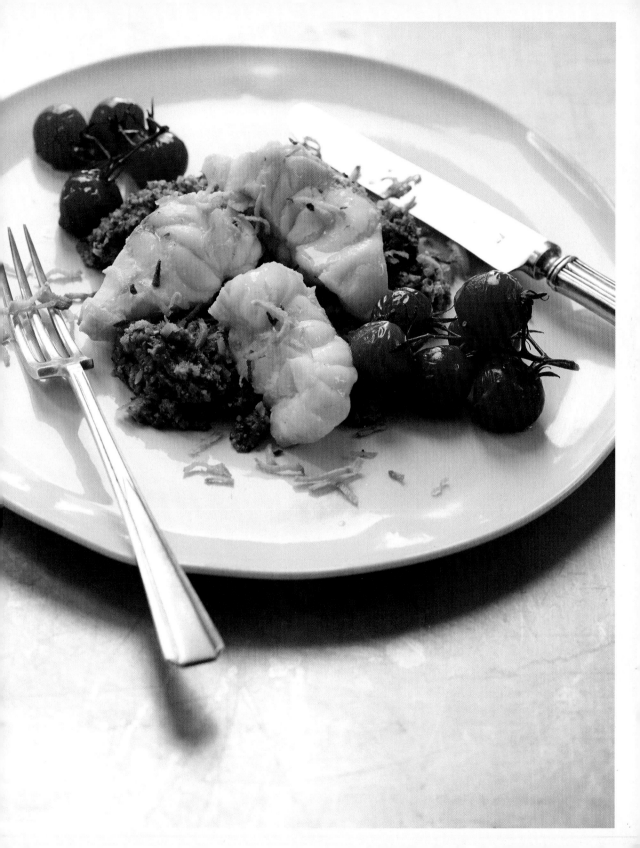

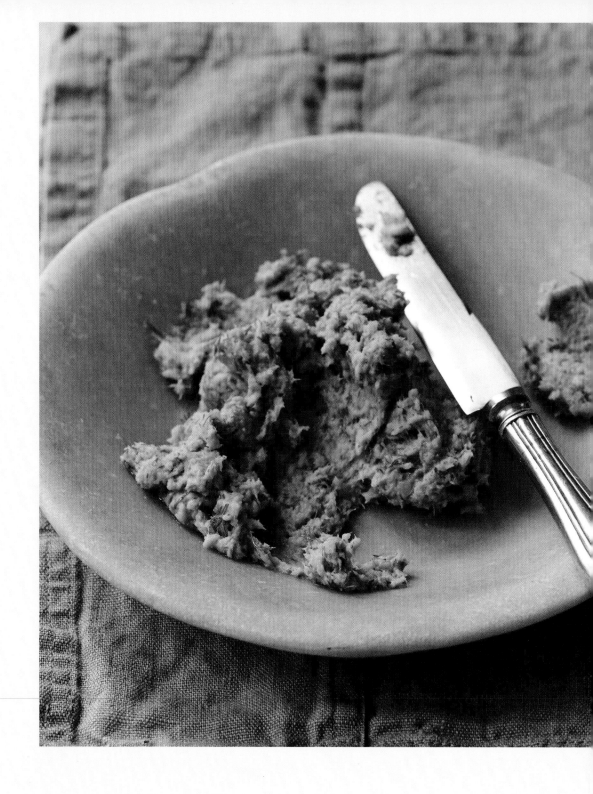

Eat. Nourish. Glow.

Smoked mackerel pâté

This works very well with natural yogurt if you are OK eating dairy.

Prep time: 5 minutes
8-oz package smoked mackerel, broken into pieces
Juice and zest of 1 lemon
A handful of fresh dill
½ avocado
Sea salt and freshly ground black pepper

Blend all the ingredients together in a mixer until combined. You may need to add a little water or extra lemon juice to taste. Serve chilled.

—Serves 2

Index &
Acknowledgments

RECIPE INDEX

263

INDEX

265

Resources

Websites

Amelia Freer FdSc, Dip ION, mBANT, mCNHC
www.freernutrition.com

Registered U.K. nutritional therapists

The British Association for Applied Nutrition and Nutritional Therapy

The Institute for Integrated Nutrition
www.integrativenutrition.com

The Institute for Functional Medicine
www.functionalmedicine.org

The Gluten Summit
www.theglutensummit.com

Coeliac U.K.

Metabolic Balance
www.metabolic-balance.com/en

The Institute for Optimum Nutrition

National Health Service U.K.

Books

Wheat Belly by William Davis M.D.

The Blood Sugar Solution by Mark Hyman M.D.

Grain Brain by David Perlmutter

Ingredients and suppliers

Freer Nutrition online Shop
www.freernutrition.com
(every product/item mentioned in the book is available here)

Bob's Red Mill
www.bobsredmill.com

Planet Organic
www.planetorganic.com

Wholefoods
www.wholefoodsmarket.com

Abel & Cole *(for organic food delivery around the U.K.)*

Biona

Coyo *(dairy free coconut yogurt)*

Coconut products
www.tiana-coconut.com

Cultured foods
www.wisechoicemarket.com/fermentedfoods

Natural Wines
www.theorganicwinecompany.com

Acknowledgments

The passion I have for nutritional therapy wouldn't burn so brightly were it not for the reward of seeing results achieved by my clients who have had faith in me and embraced my guidance over the many years I have been practicing. Without their support and recommendations to friends, family and colleagues I would not have been able to build the thriving practice I have today. They are the main source of inspiration and drive me to continue my learning in this field.

I am also grateful to my friends and colleagues in the nutritional community who have inspired and nurtured my constant quest for a better understanding for this exciting and evolving science. Without the many hours of discussing and sharing experiences, research and results with them, this book would not have been possible.

I am deeply grateful to Elizabeth Sheinkman from William Morris Endeavour, Carole Tonkinson and Vicky Eriso who gave me this opportunity to spread my nutritional principles farther afield. Thank you to the team at HarperCollins U.K., in particular Carolyn Thorne who took on the tail end of this project and gently steered me through the final stages when I became overwhelmed and fear took hold. Finally, thank you to Maria Lally who helped me give structure to my thoughts and words.

This book is dedicated to my father who died too young to learn of the path my life has taken but whom I know would have embraced everything I have written, and to mum, Justin and Paula whose unwavering love and support have made this journey possible.

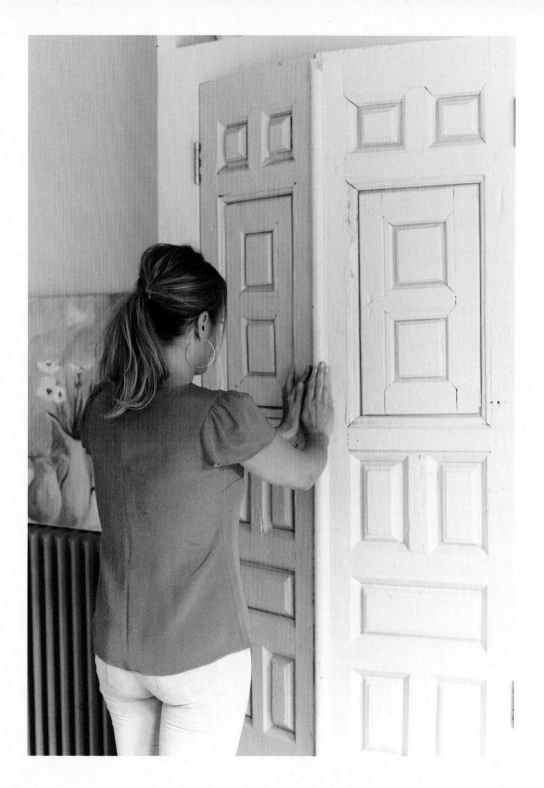

Eat. Nourish. Glow.

EAT.NOURISH.GLOW. Copyright © 2015 by Amelia Freer. All rights reserved. Printed in the United States of America. No part of this book may be used or reproduced in any manner whatsoever without written permission except in the case of brief quotations embodied in critical articles and reviews. For information, address HarperCollins Publishers, 195 Broadway, New York, NY 10007.

HarperCollins books may be purchased for educational, business, or sales promotional use. For information, please e-mail the Special Markets Department at SPsales@harpercollins.com.

Originally published in the United Kingdom in 2015 by Harper Thorsons. Originally distributed in the United States by Harper360.

Photography © 2015 by Ali Allen
Illustrations © 2015 by Heather Gatley

Library of Congress Cataloging-in-Publication Data has been applied for.

ISBN: 978-0-06-243082-3

15 16 17 18 19   NMSG/RRD   10 9 8 7 6 5 4 3 2 1